Advance praise from leading ......... ........ ....ut
*Improving Your Bedside Manner*

In an age where modern physicians have forgotten the art of medicine, choosing instead to focus on lab tests of questionable validity—and pharmaceutical company studies of even more questionable validity—Jacquelyn Small is a shining light guiding practitioners back to their healing roots. She reminds practitioners about the important things that led them into medicine in the first place, like how to care for and about their patients respectfully, and how to mobilize the patients' own ability to heal themselves—a powerful tool. After learning and applying these principles, you will become more than simply a technician. You will become the healer you were meant to be!

— Jacob Teitelbaum, MD
Medical Director, Fibromyalgia and Fatigue Centers
Author, *From Fatigued to Fantastic!*, *Three Steps to Happiness! Healing through Joy*, and *Pain Free 1-2-3: A Proven Program to Get You Pain Free*

At last, a clear, concise guide for physicians, medical students, and nurses about what really matters in that magical interaction we call the doctor-patient relationship. Any healthcare professional who aspires to become a healer instead of a mere technician should read this book.

— Larry Dossey, MD
Author, *The Extraordinary Healing Power of Ordinary Things*

*Improving Your Bedside Manner* captures the crucial factors that help people heal, that are too often neglected in professional training. This knowledge is vital not only for physicians, but nurses as well, for we spend more time at the bedside than any other healthcare professional. Highly recommended.

— Barbara Dossey, RN, PhD
Author, *Holistic Nursing: A Handbook for Practice* and
*Florence Nightengale Today: Healing, Leadership and Global Action*

Effective communication between health care professionals and those they care for is a critically important skill for the appropriate practice of medicine. *Improving Your Bedside Manner* provides the key tools necessary to enhance our natural skills as communicators and is an essential resource for all physicians and other health care professionals. In fact, what Jacquelyn Small is able to communicate in this concise work is useful for all those wanting to connect with others more deeply. Whether it is physician to patient, employer to employee, parent to child, or friend to friend, cultivating the characteristics outlined in this book will serve us all well.

— Lorenzo Cohen, PhD
Director, Integrative Medicine Program
The University of Texas M.D. Anderson Cancer Center

This is a real gem of a book! Any medical student or physician can benefit from reading it. It distills out the crucial characteristics of the most successful physicians based on research. It presents them in a way that the healer can help her or himself grow in healing potential. This book comes from both the head and the heart. It should become required reading for MDs.

— Richard P. Brown, MD
Associate Professor in Clinical Psychiatry
Columbia University College of Physicians and Surgeons

This book serves as a simple, but powerful, guide for development of the modern physician: one who is as comfortable with the patient as the technology of modern medicine. It is essential reading for every physician hoping to improve patient-centered care by incorporation of proven techniques.

The techniques discussed break down the vital but often ignored arena of patient-clinician interaction. Finally a roadmap for honestly understanding, appreciating and working with the difficult but sacred moments shared between patients and clinicians.

— Robert Alan Bonakdar, MD FAAFP
Director of Pain Management, Scripps Center
for Integrative Medicine Assistant Clinical Professor,
University of California, San Diego, School of Medicine

Jacquelyn Small discusses the often murky subject of the doctor-patient relationship in clear and humanistic terms. Her book is not just about the surface of bedside manner. It probes the forces within both the patient and the doctor that give rise to positive and negative interactions. In reading this book, medical students will learn good lessons before they acquire bad habits. Seasoned clinicians will gain awareness of the effects their behavior may be having, discover how to improve their bedside manner, and achieve better rapport with their patients. I would recommend *Improve Your Bedside Manner* to all health care providers.

— Patricia L. Gerbarg, MD
Assistant Professor in Clinical Psychiatry
New York Medical College

At the bedside between patient and physician exists a great healing opportunity and Jacquelyn Small's book lends valuable insight on how this potential can be maximized. This book is an important work for dedicated learners interested in perfecting their skills in the art of medicine.

— Roberta Lee, MD
Medical Director, Continuum Center
for Health and Healing, New York

This new book by Jacquelyn Small, *Improving Your Bedside Manner,* may be the best opportunity yet for busy physicians to consult with a communications expert whose conversational approach makes you think that you are sitting in a cozy chair in her kitchen. Small's recipes for skilled, empathic communication gleaned from her thirty plus years of experience are so simple to follow that you almost forget that bedside manner can be serious business. This book holds several keys to the establishment of comfortable, professional boundaries and effective communication techniques that will energize you, your staff, and your patients.

— Martha M. Libster, PhD, RN, CNS
Nurse Psychotherapist
Author, *Demonstrating Care: The Art of Integrative Nursing*

The content and style of what is commonly called "bedside manner" is the foundation for medical decision-making and health behavior change, yet is terribly neglected in medical education, practice, and research. Hats off to Jacquelyn Small for providing this resource for doctors to engage with and improve their manner of interacting with patients.

— Bruce Barrett, MD, PhD
Associate Professor of Family Medicine
University of Wisconsin, Madison

# IMPROVING YOUR BEDSIDE MANNER

*A Handbook for Physicians
to develop therapeutic conversations
with your patients*

*[handwritten inscription: For Wyteria — from Jacquelyn Small, In Honor of your Loving Self!]*

## JACQUELYN SMALL

*In Collaboration with Jim Mulry, MD*

Eupsychia Institute
P. O. Box 151960
Austin, TX 78715
800-546-2795
eupsychia@austin.rr.com
www.ImprovingYourBedsideManner.com


First Printing


Cataloging-in Publication Data

Small, Jacquelyn

Improving Your Bedside Manner: A handbook for
physicians to develop therapeutic conversations with your
patients

1. Physician and Patient—Interpersonal Communications
2. Medical Consultation   3. Professional Patient Relations
4. Medicine and Psychology   5. Medicine—Philosophy
I. Author   II. Title.

ISBN-10: 0-939344-22-X
ISBN-13: 978-0-939344-22-2

R 727.3 S476 2007         616.001 SM              2008900665


Printed in the United States of America
at Morgan Printing in Austin, Texas

# CONTENTS

# FOREWORD

Bedside manner is not an immediate benefit of having earned an MD degree. It involves skills, sensitivities, and interpersonal style that can and should be cultivated, however. I recommend this practical, how-to handbook as a "must read" manual for medical school and residency training in communication skills and professionalism.

Immensely thoughtful, practical, and succinctly organized, each chapter offers provocative, reflective examples of how physicians can communicate better with patients as well as improve their own self awareness. The book is helpfully divided into 10 chapters, each of which provides a definition of a specific professional communication skill, background about a professional characteristic, and provides model and "toxic" examples of how sensitive, critical clinical conversations take place.

The chapter themes cover the waterfront of what every aspiring and practicing physician needs to know to optimize their bedside manner. These qualities are respect, genuineness, empathy, warmth, self-disclosure, concreteness, immediacy, confrontation, potency, and self-actualization. This short, highly readable handbook shows how to implement these professional values and skills in a highly practical way. It does this in a heartfelt, holistic, psychologically and clinically sophisticated manner that is motivational and easy to learn.

Victor S. Sierpina, MD
Professor of Family Medicine,
University of Texas Medical Branch
W.D. and Laura Nell Nicholson
Family Professor of Integrative
Medicine, UTMB

## Acknowledgements

I am indebted to Dr. Jim Mulry for his willingness to collaborate with me on the writing of this book. His medical experience has added credibility and many examples of these traits in action in his own practice, as he is one who has an exceedingly therapeutic bedside manner and knows how to share from his heart as well as his head.

I also could never do the work I do or write the books I've written if it were not for Brenda Shea, Eupsychia's manager and my daughter. She has stood by me and held faith in this work since its inception when she was just in her teens. I know her dedication—especially to the material in this book—has touched many lives, and certainly mine.

And to the rest of my family, I melt with warmth when I think of how much you have all given me the opportunity to know what true love feels like. Mark, Tom, Brett, Michele, and my precious grandchildren, Margaret Jacquelyn and Jack Evertt—a big thank you cannot even begin to express my love and appreciation for you.

Then, finally, without all you who have come through Eupsychia's healing and training programs, I would never have developed my life's work. You are my teachers and my fellow travelers on this incredible human journey. This book is dedicated to you in gratitude and love.

# INTRODUCTION

From the beginning of the '60's through the early '80's, countless research and journal articles appeared in the field of counseling and psychotherapy indicating that regardless of your role in life—be it therapist, physician, other health provider, parent, or boss—there are 10 personality variables that determine high effectiveness as a therapeutic person in the life of another. These 10 personality traits correlate with helping as opposed to harming another person regardless of one's theoretical orientation, or the extent of your helper relationship.

In professional health care, these personal traits have been found to correlate with a wide variety of criteria of patient improvement, including psychological tests, time out of hospitals or institutions, clients' or patients' self reports, and therapist or supervisor ratings.

These 10 personality variables hold constant regardless of the diagnostic nature of your patient's problem. They have been tested with all sorts of people suffering from physical, emotional, or mental illness (1). Those who habitually remember to use these traits in their conversations with others are considered "naturally therapeutic." And the professionals who measured high in these 10 traits were found to be "high functioning" and highly sought after as therapists, doctors, mentors, and guides. Even independently, people will list these characteristics in some form when describing the type of person they would seek out when they need help.

Emerging now from this lengthy body of research, these natural "people helper" characteristics can serve as a useful guide for physicians as they start to look at themselves as therapeutic agents in the life of those they serve. They can be rapidly acquired or enhanced simply by giving them attention and practice.

Medical providers in today's world are more aware than ever that their style of relating to their patients and clients is even more vital than usual. For today, there is another body of research that correlates with these findings, specifically targeting the medical professions (2). In a research study by Dr. Howard Beckman, University of Rochester, reported in the *New York Times*, June 1, 2004, primarily only those doctors who are perceived by the patient as being arrogant, non-caring, in a hurry, or rude are hit with lawsuits when something goes wrong in their treatment of a patient. This article summarized some of these findings, with many interesting insights, such as: A psychologist at Harvard University compared the mannerisms of surgeons who had been sued multiple times with those who had never been sued and found that those with more warmth in their voices, rather than speaking with a dominant tone, were the ones never sued (3). Something even as simple as your tone of voice can make the difference in your doctor/patient relationships! The references from the popular press illustrate that these concerns are of common interest and knowledge to patients. Many practicing physicians are also paying attention.

Every physician makes mistakes, some bad enough to be considered of negligence or improper diagnostics. Unfortunately, some of this just naturally "goes with the territory" when required to be an expert on someone else's disease or critical trauma process. And, in fact, it's just human to be imperfect at anything we do. However, it has been found that patients don't file lawsuits based on the one and only criteria of medical mistakes. Most patients who suffer from serious medical errors acknowledged the mistake, but don't sue. However, those who do litigate file lawsuits because they felt rushed, ignored, or not treated like a human being by their provider who they often refer to as arrogant or cold.

Often, when more than one doctor is found to be at fault concerning a negative medical outcome, the patients don't want to sue the doctor they liked, but attempt to punish the one who was considered rude and uninterested in them. It's been found that doctors who have a caring and compassionate relationship with their patients, who actually spend 18.3 minutes versus 15 minutes with each patient during office visits, virtually never get sued! (4).

Correlating with these insights, there was an article in the *Austin American-Statesman*, Austin, in November, 2005, entitled "In patient care, empathy is the RX for ill manners, doctors learn," by *New York Times* journalist, Gina Kolata, which speaks for itself (5). Lawsuits are indeed prompted by emotional issues where the litigator is feeling betrayed or seriously harmed. And for this reason, the human side of medicine has become a major theme in today's medical journals and conventions. And it's no wonder, really, when we remember that it's humans that we serve!

I believe we all know that when we're in a life crisis of any kind, being in the presence of someone who is empathic, who listens and really cares, we feel better afterward. And even perhaps our health improves. As a long-time psychotherapist and teacher of therapeutic processes, I've found this to be consistently the truth, sometimes almost to a miraculous degree. As Dr. Candace Pert's research concerning the biochemical links

15

between consciousness, mind and body, indicates so poignantly, there is no way we can separate emotional well-being from physical health: they go hand-in-hand to bring us health or illness (6). The mind/body medicine field is replete today with facts proving that our emotional life feeds our physical health to a dramatic degree, noted especially in cancer and heart attack survivors.

So if you are a physician or other medical provider reading this book, you may be hoping to improve your relationships with your patients. And if so, you will benefit very quickly from a thorough examination and understanding of these traits-in-action. And the good news is: You already have these natural human qualities built within your psyche, so you don't have to go out seeking them in long hours of study and training. With only a few hours of focus, and a willingness to practice with your patients, you can learn to bring forth that which is already within you in a highly therapeutic manner. And you can do this, not in some awkward or uncomfortable "pretend" manner, but by still just naturally being yourself.

I know how valuable every minute of your time is. In today's medical morass of managed care, where you are needing to increase the numbers of patients you see each day to bill for insurance, it's crucial that you learn to improve your bedside manner to its ultimate capability—and as quickly and easily as possible, not only for your patients' well-being, but also to ease your mind from lawsuit threats.

This little book is not a simple recipe book for knowing *about* these traits. It's a "knowing in your bones" reminder of what naturally helps rather than hinders others in our verbal exchanges with them. Anyone can memorize by rote a given set of techniques, but the key to any therapeutic relating lies in the mystery of the therapeutic relationship itself. Somewhere within the physician and one's patient something unites and creates a sense of deep compassion and desire to truly be there for another, resulting in the patient feeling "heard."

The renowned family therapist, Dr. Nathan Ackerman, claims that, like medicine itself, therapeutic relating is not a skill, but an art—that being a therapeutic helper is *a way of being* rather than a set of learned techniques. The question then becomes: Can something as artistic, powerful, mysterious, and creative as "therapeutic relating" be taught as skill development? Or are some of us just born with this ability while others are not? If being therapeutic is dependent upon such ill-defined phrases as "a total way of being," what on earth can we attempt to teach?

In looking over these naturally therapeutic characteristics that have emerged from the much less mystical world of empirical research, we can see quickly that these qualities break down into three categories of relating: five are supportive traits, three are challenging, and two are "total way of being" qualities.

If you feel weak in any of the supportive or challenging traits, reading this book and then practicing the ones you're less comfortable with will bring them forth more naturally. However, the two most powerful and advanced "total way of being" traits, Potency and Self-actualization, are qualities of your selfhood that must be cultivated through your own healing and personal work on yourself, and might require a total transformation of your familiar way of relating.

Based on my 33 years of training counselors and other health professionals and Dr. Jim's 30 years of medical practice, including six years as an assistant professor in a medical school, here's our answer: Just as an acorn has the one and only innate potential to become an oak tree, just by naturally being ourselves, we all have the inherent ability to be compassionate, creative and authentic in our unique expression. We simply have to remove the blocks in attitude, caused by our own unhealed issues that may be keeping us from being fully ourselves. While some have farther to go, all of us can markedly improve.

When practiced in your relationships with your patients day in and day out, gradually learning when to bring forth each of these therapeutic traits, you will change and grow along with those you serve. And everyone in your intimate life will notice these changes with admiration—and frankly, often with much relief! You probably don't realize that as physicians, you may have been humorously referred to for years as an "M.Diety" behind your back. Or you will hear the joke: Do you know the difference between God and a doctor? And the answer is, God knows he's not a doctor.

We do so often blame doctors for being arrogant "know-it-alls." And yet, isn't it true that we *want* our doctors to know everything there is to know about our particular disease and how to cure it? We certainly don't want to hear "I'm sorry, I just don't know anything about this" and then be charged $90 for the 15-minute office visit! So I believe we all need to become more compassionate with one another—doctors and patients alike—and honor the medical profession for its undying commitment to our critical life and death issues.

We must all realize that physicians are trained to dis-identify as much as possible with human suffering, to remain objective and keep their hearts defended when dealing with the grief surrounding the seriously ill and dying. The fear is they might become too emotionally overwhelmed to be effective at times when it's crucial that they be so. However, avoiding the human tendency to paralysis or overreaction to pain has its price when overdone. In fact, the research underlying this material shows quite dramatically that in many of the helping professions—and certainly evident in the medical world—we have had *trained out* of us our most natural therapeutic skills. One study even revealed that the higher the academic degree, the less therapeutic the helper was (7). The paradoxical result is that the most therapeutic person in one's life sometimes turns out to be one's hairdresser or bartender! Western medicine has made great scientific advances since Hippocrates rejected the mystical origin of disease. Some have carried empiricism too far. So, as a profession, we are now moving from biomedicine to a biopsychosocial model, hoping to become more holistic in our approach.

Dr. Jim notes the high price physicians pay for the drive that allows them to complete an extra decade of schooling and then to work day and night, often without real patient gratitude and recently with decreasing compensation. The denial system that leads physicians to do this, he says, results in excessive rates of divorce, suicide, and addiction, suggesting that their self-awareness is not always fully developed. When teaching at the medical school, he participated in one survey that found that at least 40% of the medical students came from troubled, usually alcoholic families, which seemed to have induced self denial and self deception as well as high compensating energy.

As a physician, you know that nearly everyday you are required to be present and totally alert right when a patient or family member is undergoing the most serious, life-threatening issues they may ever face —where fear, grief, broken hearts, disappointment, rage, and bitterness climb to their ultimate feeling states. So naturally, you've had to learn to sometimes close your heart in order to maintain objectivity and technical competence. Yet, it's clearly no wonder that lawsuits are the result when someone has felt ignored, talked down to, or downright insulted by a doctor with a superior attitude. You are the one—and sometimes the only one—who can offer real hope, compassion, and a sense of inner strength for the one sitting on your examining table, or for the family member hearing the devastating news.

It's time now to bring this simple, clear, and potent knowledge to you, to assist you in your vital work of healing and saving lives, in the least amount of your valuable time possible. In this short handbook, we will quickly define each personality characteristic, and give you examples of how each one sounds *in vivo* with a patient. We will also offer examples of what I term "toxic relating," which is the absence of these traits in action. Then, in a brief discussion of each, you can determine for yourself which of these traits you might lack, or fail to use, or those you already naturally use. This is a self-diagnostic, easy way for you to grow and evolve in your profession.

# How to Use This Book

These natural characteristics you already possess! We will explore in detail each one so that you may recognize them in yourself and know when and how to use them. They are: Empathy, Genuineness, Respect, Self-disclosure, Warmth, Immediacy, Concreteness, Therapeutic Confrontation, Potency and Self-actualization.

Eight of these personality variables we'll explore are either supportive, rapport-building traits, or they help us therapeutically confront our patients in an effective, caring manner, reminding them that in order to heal they must come out of denial and take responsibility for their part in their healing process. Since you already possess these characteristics, these eight human relational skills can be easily utilized with little need for long hours of training, which is good news for you as a busy physician. You only need to be reminded you have them and learn when and how to express them in your conversations with your patients and their family members. Or, when you find yourself in trouble in a patient relationship, you can check to see which of these traits was absent and seek to correct the error.

As mentioned earlier, the final two therapeutic traits found in high-functioning therapists —Potency and Self-actualization—are the higher *being level* characteristics you can gain only through personal work on yourself and conscious experience in living. These two, you must evolve into through personal commitment to your own growth and transformation.

After each exemplary dialogue, we have added short discussions and explanations of the dynamics involved in each particular interaction described, pointing out what made it therapeutic or toxic, and what traps to watch out for.

Each therapeutic variable will be defined and you can study the dialogue given that offers you an example of how each variable sounds in a doctor/patient conversation. We will also give you an example of a toxic dialogue, where this therapeutic trait is absent. Through self-analysis, you can determine which traits you are already highly developed in and which ones you may need to make more conscious and remind yourself to use. Usually, you are better at the rapport-building traits or the confrontational ones, depending on your particular personality style.

It's my conviction that good therapeutic training can simply involve a mere "letting go" again and being naturally your openhearted self. Dr. Jim and I offer this information to you, with love.

*A Note about Gender.* No bias toward gender is intended here. I will be using examples of dialogues with both male and female doctors to avoid the awkwardness of saying "he or she" over and over. And Dr. Jim will be speaking from his own case studies.

# IMPROVING YOUR BEDSIDE MANNER

# Chapter One

# Respect

Definition. Noticing with considerate attention the views and feelings of another with an attitude of high regard for every person, even those who differ greatly from you in culture, lifestyle, or habits.

Description. In conversations with one's patients, this is the physician's ability to communicate to his patient his sincere belief that every person is an equal and has the inherent strength and capacity to live a meaningful life, with the right to choose one's own alternatives and make one's own decisions.

Respect is a supportive, rapport-building personality trait that leads to good self-feeling and trust in those we help. To bring forth this natural human quality, you must be willing to become a sensitive listener to your patient. Here's an example of what it would look like in conversation with a patient:

**Respect-in-action:**

Patient: "I know you want me to take these anti-depressants. But frankly, I'm not much on using pharmaceutical drugs of any kind. Do you know of an herbal remedy or something more natural that might work for my sensitive body instead?"

Doctor: "Let me get back to you on that. I'll have to do a little research, just to make sure we use something really known to be effective. I appreciate the fact that your body is sensitive to drugs. And I'll do this quickly, as I realize you are suffering.

Here, the doctor respects this client's feeling of knowing her own body, and even though quite busy, is willing to help her find an alternative solution that is sound. Also the physician does not denigrate her desire to use an alternative approach. This is a therapeutic response that builds upon the patient's sense of value and confidence. Though there is still no solution to what she may need to feel better, she will leave the doctor's office feeling better about herself.

Trained and constantly updating in high-tech, disease-oriented medicine, most doctors are not educated in some of the newer, more alternative methods of healing that many patients today are learning about. Many people today want to be an active participant in their health care and hope to have a nurturing, collaborative relationship with their caregivers. In this dialogue, this need is honored, even though the doctor still may decide after researching it that the patient may need some form of conventional medical treatment.

Here's another therapeutic response to this patient, using Respect:

Doctor: I truly do not know of a good alternative. But that's not to say there isn't one out there. With your sensitivities, you might be well served by seeing Dr. Chang who is a specialist in herbal remedies. She is trained in both Chinese and Western medicine and I have a great deal of respect for her. And I will be glad to collaborate with her on a treatment plan, with your permission.

In this response, the doctor isn't afraid to reveal that he doesn't have all the answers, and is letting this patient know he's willing to help her find what she is seeking in her own way. This response is high in Respect, as it honors the patient's own interest in alternative approaches, even though this physician is not schooled in herbal medicine. This type of communication equalizes the relationship.

And from Dr. Jim, we get this clinical example that is highly respectful and with a satisfactory medical outcome:

He remembers many patients who had been on pharmaceutical thyroid replacement, which contains only one of two main thyroid hormones. These patients felt unwell and asked to change to a more natural product. He says that he explained the natural product contained a balanced mix of the two hormones, but was also chemically less standardized, and, therefore theoretically less predictable and less medically desirable. In one case, the patient and Dr. Jim agreed to try the natural product for a period of time. Later tests consistently showed the condition was well controlled and the patient is still reporting being happy, feeling much better, and very satisfied with the medical encounter.

**Toxic Responses:**

Doctor: I haven't got time to research anything like this. All this alternative stuff is questionable anyway. You'd do better just to do as I say so you can start feeling better. That's the goal, isn't it? You need to feel better. And these pharmaceutical antidepressants are the only proven treatment.

This response shows a complete lack of respect for the patient's wishes or knowledge of her own body. This response also ignores the science that reveals most antidepressants help two-thirds of patients, but the placebo in the study helps one-half of the controls. The drug affect is only 15%! The doctor is not really open to hearing her real concern based on her own experience about how drugs affect her body. He is, instead, more invested in being right, with the attitude that she has no right to question his authority. And further, he is putting her down for believing that some herbal remedy might have value, when, really, he just lacks education on the subject.

Any response that puts down the patient's own needs and knowledge of her body would be anti-therapeutic. Ideally, the doctor respectfully provides a balance by offering scientific knowledge, and the patient contributes their knowledge of themselves. Even if the patient's wishes are medically implausible, you are getting valuable information about her belief system and desires for ways to heal. It's crucial to one's healing process to find out what motivates your patients and what gives them passion.

We must never forget that the life force itself is what does the healing. When one lacks the desire to live or be well, the battle may well be lost.

Reflect on how you might draw more personal information from your patients in the short time you have with them, about their interests and motivations for a healthy life. Practitioners often have only 10 to 15 minutes to interview, clarify, examine, organize, plan, prescribe and document a patient, and this is a major problem, so that listening with patience is challenging.

And if a diagnosis has sounded vague or not thoroughly understood by your patient, be willing to speak in plain language about what her main problem is, what she can do to help, and why.

And remember, using too much medical jargon is also disrespectful, as it is often indecipherable, or even frightening to your patients. So be sure and speak in ordinary language as much as possible when giving your patients their test results or medical diagnoses.

## And Here Are Some Traps:

Many patients have toxic lifestyles or personalities and blindly sabotage themselves with such obvious and self destructive patterns that their complaints can seem almost farcical and activate the providers' personal issues, such as need for authority or compliance. You can reflect on this and see if this ever applies to you.

You can always respectfully discuss each specific situation with your patients, allowing them to choose the level of medical involvement they prefer.

## *Self-reflection:*

Ask yourself if you are the type of person who has the need to always be right, or never questioned. Do you become defensive when someone differs with you about something in your field of specialty? Do you argue, or abruptly shut down conversations where you might be called upon to say, "I don't know" or, "You may be right." Be honest with yourself about this. And if you realize this is an issue for you, ask yourself where does your need to be right come from? What is your fear of being questioned? Perhaps you had parents or other significant adults in your childhood who would not allow you to make mistakes.

How do you feel about the fact that your patients are getting more sophisticated in their knowledge of their own health issues? Is it acceptable for you to realize your patients today want more time with you to dialogue medical options, or seek more emotional support? This is a difficult transition to make from the old paradigm, a more authoritarian labeling and disease model of medicine.

This shift in paradigms, from being the outside expert to patients wishing to collaborate more in their own intelligent medical choices, is happening at the same time managed care and insurance companies expect you to increase your patient-load and spend less time with each patient. Doctors who never get sued do spend a few more minutes with each patient than those physicians who tend to get sued—just a few more minutes makes a difference. Food for thought.

# CHAPTER TWO

# Genuineness

DEFINITION: Genuineness describes one's sincere authenticity and willingness to be oneself.

DESCRIPTION: This trait marks the ability for the physician to behave in non-phony, non-role-playing, and non-defensive ways. There is no discrepancy between one's words and outer behaviors with one's inner feelings.

## Genuineness-in-action:

Patient: (shuddering and fighting back tears) "I'm so scared. . . just terrified, in fact. I know you haven't given me a death sentence. But with this type of cancer, I know my chances are very slim. What can I do to make it go away? I can't believe this is happening to me."

Doctor: (leaning toward her patient) Well. . . . Gosh, Mary, I wish I had a magic answer for you. (softly) I'm so sorry this is happening. I can't give you any kind of absolute medical guarantee about the outcome here. We just have to work together with all the medical magic and faith we can muster. This is the hardest part of my job: seeing you so deeply hurt and scared. I *can* promise you this: I will work with everything we know to help you feel better and, hopefully, to heal. Even though the research isn't on our side here, we have seen some cases where this type of cancer goes into spontaneous remission with treatment. Whenever you feel ready, please ask your husband to come in with you and we'll talk over our next step together.

Dr. Jim recalls a patient with severe ovarian cancer with partial responses, but much toxicity from multiple rounds of chemo. Her question to me was is it worth it to be fighting? Knowing that she had previously successfully fought through some severe illnesses and still had a small chance of recovery, I helped her to continue her own basic lifelong value of struggling for success, by taking another round of treatment.

She was comfortable with this after my reassurance that I would tell her directly and immediately if at any time her situation had become completely hopeless. I believe my genuineness and faith in her willingness to heal helped her get better.

In both these examples, the physician has made a sincere, frank statement of authenticity, not forced but arising naturally. In each dialogue the patient will feel heard with a sense that her doctor is a real person who truly cares and who is telling her the complete truth.

In the first example, not only the doctor's words, but her body language, too, indicate her real feelings about this tragic health diagnosis that may indeed be hopeless in terms of a cure. Yet, she indicates she is willing to do everything in her power to help her patient not suffer, physically or emotionally. And further, she is open to helping the husband become involved in his wife's care as well.

Dr. Jim so beautifully demonstrates how validating a patient's inner strengths from past knowledge and also using his own faith to elicit his patient's faith is the healing factor here.

These doctor/patient conversations lead to deepening the rapport between the doctor and the patient—which will be so crucial if the patient is indeed entering into a death process. In the first example, the doctor wasn't afraid to say she feels sad. And this is a bit unusual for a physician to say, as most medical training teaches that feelings are not to be shared with a patient. But ask yourself: What is the natural human response? It's sorrow, of course—and angst about the possible negative outcome. Also, feelings of helplessness will often accompany a human crisis like this.

Being genuinely heartfelt with patients is a very confusing issue for many professional health care providers. Being oneself never has to violate one's professionalism. Good judgment is needed, of course. But being genuine in your natural human responses to those in need brings therapeutic trust and relief. Perhaps we'll never know for certain, but it could be that emotional wellness and a strong sense of being loved and cared for just might be what leads to those mysterious spontaneous remissions! More research is needed in this crucial area of the emotional/physical connection. We do already know that people who have had a heart attack and feel loved have less second heart attacks than those who have no one in their lives to care deeply for them. And cancer patients with a positive attitude and positive coping skills are better able to keep their immune systems active than are those who feel helpless and despairing.

**Toxic Response:**

Doctor: (hurriedly) "Yes, yes. I know how it feels. Let's move on with your treatment plan. . . that needs to start immediately, by the way. And don't worry. We're going to do all we can."

Though this doctor seems to be trying to be positive, this response can be experienced as impatience—maybe due to her heavy schedule—or that she is uncomfortable with emotion. This type of response would reinforce the patient's defenses against feeling the natural fear and pain associated with this life-threatening diagnosis. It moves her away from her real experience of the moment in a distance-keeping, task-oriented discussion. And this is happening at a time when she really needs to feel the emotional support from her physician. Also, it lacks credibility to hear the doctor say, "I know how it feels." Does she really know how this feels? Probably not, unless there has been a similar diagnosis occurring in the doctor's own personal life.

This patient will leave this appointment feeling emotionally blocked, discounted and "put aside." And right at a time when she really needs a close professional involvement with her primary medical caregiver, the only person she can count on to maybe even save her life.

Physicians are trained to remain in their professional role and stay objective while working with patients. And this is certainly understandable and useful for technical aspects of treatment and for objectivity. And there are times, especially with certain types of patients, when this stance is exactly the correct approach. As one example, doctors regularly review treatment for themselves or family members with other physician colleagues, to maintain objectivity. For another example, some patients can become too needy and demanding for a doctor's constant primary attention, when their medical issues truly do not require such attention. With too much encouragement, some will even call the doctor at home too often, signaling a state of overdependence.

However, there comes a time when this kind of professional attitude can sound cold and too aloof to be therapeutic. Perhaps sometimes the doctor himself is defending against emotional pain. Balance is ideal when coupled with a strong sense of good judgment and willingness to look at oneself. This issue of genuine relating with a personal "feel" to it needs to be examined by every physician.

### And Here Are Some Traps:

Realizing one's personal tendency to overreact often triggers a response of repression. Stuffing feelings allows more negative emotional build up and eventually more outbursts. A better strategy would be to talk through the emotions or issues with a friend or colleague when the emotionally charged issues are still small, rather than believing you're not to "make waves." Trying to avoid the internal build-up by repressing feelings can eventually blindside you by some unexpected and inappropriate release.

Genuine empathy in some situations can bring up the doctor's own active emotional issues, which can elicit an avoidance reaction. This causes the patient to feel dismissed. Physicians can learn to listen for the possibility of personal issues surfacing and separate them from the patient interaction.

Alternatively, some patients want the doctor to be an idealized parent, lover or soul mate. Unfortunately, being put "on a pedestal" creates patient expectations that are quite unrealistic and often lead to a sense of betrayal when the doctor is unresponsive to a romantic seduction or is proven to have "clay feet."

This happens in my counseling experience with clients as well. And I try to nip in the bud any idolizing of me by sharing some of my own foibles, letting them see that I am just as imperfect a human as anyone. With this awareness, physicians can learn to directly avoid the patient's excessive expectations in a similar fashion. Just being yourself is a wonderful antidote for this type of transference that can become exceedingly harmful if not addressed.

### Transference and Counter-Transference

Transference is a very prominent and often harmful dynamic that occurs between doctors and their patients. The same happens with ministers, therapists, teachers, or anyone in a "savior" or "mentor" role. This dynamic can turn into strong feelings of being romantically in love with one's "savior" or "high priest." This is called transference. Counter-transference is the dynamic that occurs when the physician or mentor feels romantic toward a patient, student, or parishioner. Counter-transference feelings should never be shared with anyone seeking your help or looking up to you—not in any way whatsoever. You need to process these feelings in the safe container of a therapy session, or with a friend or family member you can absolutely trust to hold the confidence. Even your body language and voice intonation must be carefully monitored to show no sign of flirtation or willingness to indulge, because a patient like this will look for *any* possible hint that you might return these feelings. And then the fantasy heightens, and you may have a real mess on your hands.

Learning to deal with transference and counter-transference issues therapeutically is intricate and "tricky," but can also be very therapeutic if handled consciously. You don't want to put down your patient or client for the feelings he or she may be having toward you. Yet, at the same time you must be absolutely clear that you are not available for any kind of flirtation or intimate involvement.

Here's what a therapeutic response can sound like if a patient ever declares having fallen in love with you, or begins to behave in overtly obvious seductive or sexual ways:

Doctor: Libby, you are an attractive woman and deserve to have a wonderful, loving mate in your life. I am very honored that you see me in such a positive light, and I really do care for you as your physician. But you need to know that I'm completely in love with my wife and am not open to any kind of romance with anyone else. That door is closed. Let's just remember I am your doctor and you are my patient. And let's get on with getting your health better. (friendly smile, informal attitude) How's that? This *is* our right relationship.

And if the patient then goes into an emotional reaction and starts crying, blaming, or feeling hurt, you can listen for a while in a genuinely caring, non-reactive manner. But after a few minutes, you may need to tell this patient quite honestly that you are not a therapist, and you sense that she may really need to see someone to help her work through this issue.

As a former Protective Services social worker, I remind you here that the two groups of people who abuse children the most severely are the military and the religious. This points to a need for more heart feeling—more openness, emotional availability, and compassion in raising our children with more conscious awareness concerning their discipline, safety, and emotional needs. Patients who implore you to love them inappropriately are often from these abusive families and seek out doctors for special attention. They are vulnerable to rejection and even to suicide when a "god" rejects them. So be careful in this regard. Your open heart with appropriate boundaries are essential to this person's well-being.

### *Self-reflection:*

People who decide to be physicians or some type of health care provider are often from families that are either very intellectual and don't allow much feeling to be expressed. Or, they are from dysfunctional families and their desire to serve is also a way of helping themselves.

If you see that you are terribly uncomfortable with feelings, and have even been given feedback that your intimates cannot relate to you emotionally, then ask yourself: When did I shut down my heart? What kind of childhood did I have? What attitude was I imprinted with about the importance of having genuine, appropriate feelings? How was I punished as a child? And what was I punished for? What kind of role models did I have growing up in this regard?

Where do you stand in all this? Perhaps you realize you are even too heartfelt and open with your clients. If so, you will need to practice some of the more challenging, concrete skills we'll study later. If you feel imbalanced in either direction— either too heartfelt and open, or too demanding and "militaristic," make a vow to work on yourself and see if more balance can come into your way of being. Practicing the skills you feel weak in while face to face with your patients will go a long way.

As mentioned in the Introduction, you may be more natural with the heartfelt, rapport-building personality qualities, or better at the more concrete or confrontational ones. If you were raised by parents who never touched you or rarely showed emotion (except perhaps strong temper when you didn't mind them), you may have been imprinted with extreme feelings of discomfort when in an emotionally-laden situation. If so, you will have developed a psychological defense that squashes your own emotional responses in life, either by withdrawing, re-directing, or shutting down the interaction.

In cases like this, these natural emotional responses felt throughout one's life have had to go somewhere. They land in one's subconscious state of being and frankly, can paralyze your feeling nature, or burst out in extreme rage, or in some other inappropriate ways when some outside person or event triggers the pent-up issue.

Dr. Jim recalls that he used to experience emotional numbness during a medical crisis, or other emotional situations—a condition called Alexethymia. He would not have real feelings for one to two days after an emergency. Now this can be a real asset in the calm technical response needed in a medical crisis, but a serious liability at other times. Both in routine medical care and at home with his family, Dr. Jim says he needed to learn to experience emotions. He also says that the strategies in this book have greatly improved this situation for him.

We really don't want to live our lives without feeling. It leads to our own ill health and goodness knows, it subtracts all the joy from life. And certainly, it can inhibit or destroy our ability to be in intimate, trustworthy relationships with our spouses, children, parents, and closest friends, as well as appropriate openness and warmth with our patients and staff. A good physician will model emotional health along with the need for physical wellness.

Reflect for a moment of whether you are more comfortable opening your heart and being soft and kind with your patients. Or are you more at ease when needing to discipline them or correct what you perceive as their poor attitude, decisions, or behavior? Neither is wrong. Both skills are needed in any kind of effective people work.

# Chapter Three

# Empathy

DEFINITION: The capacity for participating in, or having a vicarious experience of, another's feelings, volitions, or ideas in both content and context.

DESCRIPTION: Empathy has two aspects to it in a conversation: It marks the ability to perceive or "feel" another's experience and then to communicate that perception back to the individual so that they feel heard. Here's an example of what it would look like *in vivo:*

**Empathy-in-action:**

Patient: (head down, arms crossed over heart in a constricted manner) I know this stress is killing me. I just can't take much more of this taking care of two sick parents. They're both demanding so much from me and don't even know they're doing it. My nerves are shot.

Doctor: Goodness me, Jonathan, I can tell you're struggling just to breathe! My heart really goes out to you. I know this is a very difficult time in your life. It does sound to me like your family is smothering you with all this pressure to meet their needs. . . *and* you must be feeling a sense of hopelessness that it will ever end.

This empathic statement is open-ended and invites the patient to talk more about his issue with his parents, which is helpful to be able to vent with someone he can trust. Notice how the doctor focused the conversation on his patient's feelings in that moment rather than talking about the medical treatment for stress. This is a caring response that makes the client feel heard.

People who rate high in Empathy are good at hearing what's really being said at the non-verbal level, what's beneath the surface of the content they are expressing. The doctor in this dialogue had noticed his patient's body language and tone of voice as well as the content of the problem, and responded on that level to both the dialogue and nonverbal clues that spoke the hopelessness the doctor picked up on.

Oftentimes, an empathic statement usually begins with "I feel. . . " or "I sense. . . " rather than "You are. . . ." or "You need to. . . ." "You" statements can sound judgmental or cold and insincere, whereas "I" statements contain both a genuine self-disclosure and often true Empathy. You'll see later that Self-disclosure is another of the therapeutic variables that correlate with high effectiveness as a therapeutic helper. Statements like "Gosh, I *felt* that as you said it, because I've been in this situation in my life. I know how it feels."

**Toxic Responses:**

Doctor: You don't need to stress so much about this. You just have to learn to detach a little more. Lots of people wind up having to care for their aging parents. The way you handle this is you make the best of it till their time comes.

And since you don't have other siblings close by, this duty is simply going to fall mostly on you. That's just the way it is. Moaning about it doesn't help at all, because you know you're going to do all that's required for them right now. So just do it."

Now, even though the doctor is fully engaging here, and everything he says in this response is no doubt the truth—even to the point that he's helping create balance to the patient's over-reaction—this approach lacks Empathy. It will more than likely produce guilt and even more feelings of pressure, rather than any sense of emotional support, or of feeling heard. Also, this response is a "door closer" to any more dialogue with this physician, and will shut the patient down with a warning that it's not safe to talk to about this problem here. Instead of building rapport with this patient, it has shattered it.

Often, we make the error of having ready-made answers to people who are "in process"—or in the *working through* stage—about a difficult situation. "You've really got a pretty good life. Remember the people starving in Darfur." Or, "Oh, I hear this all the time from people with aging parents. It's just part of life." So, in other words, "Get over it." Right? And don't we wish we could just get over all our difficult life situations! But it doesn't work that way, does it? When a fearful or negative feeling enters our bodies, it's there to be dealt with realistically. It can't be placated or repressed. If it went in, it's somehow going to need to come out, and hopefully, therapeutically. This is where Empathy comes in.

In therapy, we always know the way out is *through*. Specifically, the experience and the verbal expression of the emotion must be made conscious and expressed. Without a safe container for working through our emotional upsets, we repress them and thereby set up conditions for more upsets and eventually more stress induced physical pain and disease.

Any response we use that replies with generalities about "all the people in the world," discounts a person's personal feelings about an individual life situation. At times like these, we don't relate to "all the people in the world;" our problem feels very personal and unique. So we need a personal response to move toward any kind of relevant solution or healing.

People who rate high in Empathy are natural good listeners and can hear what's really being said beneath the surface of the content they are expressing. Therapists often speak of the difference between "content" and "process," and respond as much as possible to the non-verbal process underneath the content. We don't discount the content, but it's the process that usually needs addressing.

### And Here Are Some Traps:

Doctors have told me they fear being drawn into doing therapy with their patients, both for lack of time and also for lack of skill in such matters. I understand this. And it's not necessary that you become a therapist to be an empathic listener. In fact, the more empathic you learn to be, the quicker you can establish rapport and say therapeutic things to your patients in the shortest amount of time.

So study the types of responses demonstrated above, and see if your own inner wisdom won't awaken to bring forth your own natural Empathy for those is pain.

We may find ourselves over- or under-reacting to noncompliant patients. And this issue may be our own. If you truly feel incapable of having heart to heart conversations with your patients, or know that you remain overly distant, you may want to consider adding another person to the treatment team. Often a Physician's Assistant can serve this valuable purpose.

A second trap is to personally project one's own emotion onto the patient, then demand that the patient respond as you believe you would act in the same situation. We may have a habit of living in a rather "narcissistic bubble" with the unexamined belief that other people think and feel about things exactly the same way we do. Or if not, they should!

Another trap is the patient may use words that don't convey the real meaning of what she's attempting to communicate. Dr. Jim well remembers a stoic patient who said only "I hurt" with no expression and complete refusal to use any pain medicine. What this patient meant was "I am suffering terribly or I would not disclose this at all." When an unanticipated and unavoidable complication of her treatment developed, she felt so misunderstood and betrayed that she actually sued. Although the suit was unsuccessful, Dr. Jim feels his lack of alertness to the hidden message destroyed their relationship and led to a long process for successful self-defense.

### Self-reflection:

Take a moment to reflect on your usual way of speaking with your patients. . . . Are you a natural good listener who feels an empathic connection to your patients when they are suffering emotionally? Or do you seek to shut down the emotions as quickly as possible, feeling uncomfortable about any show of emotion?

Your feeling states are what connect you to life, not just the painful parts, but to the joyful, even blissful ones, as well. Feelings are one! And as earlier mentioned, if you consistently shut off the negative feelings, you are also limiting your ability to feel joy.

Ask yourself what kinds of feelings you may be resisting in your own relationships? What kind of feedback do you get from those close to you? Perhaps a spouse is often saying that you are not "there" emotionally. And if so, are you willing to look at this and attempt to rectify this paucity that may exist in your emotional life? Maybe somewhere down the line you were given the idea that having emotions is weak. If so, you have a void in your own way of being in the world fully and completely. Learning to control your emotional reactions may have saved you as a child if you were punished for expressing feelings. But now, today, as a health provider and perhaps a family member, too, you might benefit greatly by doing some emotional healing work of your own. When our emotions are balanced and healthy, we live with an open heart. Then, it's almost impossible to lack Empathy in our meaningful conversations.

# CHAPTER FOUR

# Warmth

DEFINITION: The quality or state of being warm and open-hearted in one's reception of another.

Description: Warmth is often demonstrated non-verbally in communication with your patients. Behaviors such as smiles, the looks on your face, leaning forward in an interested, involved manner when your patient is speaking, and other natural human responses are evidence of this characteristic. Tone of voice can also feel warm or cold and aloof.

In the research concerning this personality variable, therapists who rated high in warmth were very spontaneous with their body movements, at home in their bodies and feelings, and not afraid to show deep caring in many non-verbal expressions. Therapists who were rigid, detached, and unresponsive to emotion were less able to establish rapport with their clients. Consequently, clients often terminated the relationship prematurely, or failed to show up for appointments.

As a means to convey this trait in non-emergency office calls, Dr. Jim expresses his genuine pleasure in seeing the patient again, shaking hands with a smile and welcoming them back to the office.

**Warmth-in-action:**

Patient: (trembling voice) Ever since my husband left, I've not been able to sleep. (slumping in her chair and fidgeting with her fingers) I need some medicine to help me. But I worry about getting addicted to prescription drugs. I want so badly to get over these awful feelings of fear and despair. I'm so glad I have a good doctor like you who understands.

Doctor: Karen, your feelings are so natural, and there are some medicines I can recommend to help you. I'll be right here for you as you go through this. (voice tone is soft and comforting). We can use medications for a while, and then help you find deeper ways to heal this loss of your marriage. (getting up from his chair and light-heartedly pulling her up by her hands) Now, come on, let's get this exam over with!

On the surface, this may seem to be too intimate a contact between a male physician and his female patient. But it's not inappropriate in this context. This patient has been under the care of this physician for over two years. So they know each other well. And nothing in his tone or behavior has an inappropriate or sexual quality to it. It is simply a heartfelt response to a patient in deep grief and fear. This is a therapeutic interchange where the healing agent is the quality of Warmth.

Direct service workers in any form of health care have always known that clean and clear physical touch is therapeutic. Yet, we also know that doctors are very careful how and when to touch their patients for fear of misunderstood motive, or even of being sued. So each of you reading this need to decide for yourself how you feel about touching your clients when it's simply the normal, obvious thing to do. There is an enormous difference in heartfelt touch and sexual "come ons." We can all "feel" or sense when it's not clean. Following well-intentioned instincts is often a great guide as long as no unconscious personal issues exist to surface.

If your motives have nothing whatsoever to do with physical attraction or need, then you are absolutely appropriate to sometimes touch your client in ways anyone just naturally would. For example, sometimes a patient will spontaneously reach out and give you a hug. Or, if both are sitting, might pat you on the knee, or grab your hand during an emotional expression of some kind. To react as though you are abruptly pulling away can be more of a sign of fear of one's response than simply allowing the natural heartfelt touch to occur.

Also, as you study these natural human traits, you will see how they all merge together as just our way of being when we are naturally caring and helpful. If it is simply not a genuine response for you to ever touch a client or be openhearted with them, you needn't become "phony" in your desire to improve your rapport-building skills. Authenticity is Genuineness-in-action and must never be violated because this is what builds trust. You may be more formal, dignified and reserved in your natural personality, so that any kind of touch other than a handshake feels unnatural for you. If so, being high functioning in Empathy and Genuineness will be enough.

**Toxic Responses:**

Doctor: Well, (getting up from his chair) we need to get on with your examination. Let's get to it here, and see how you're doing physically.

Or, often, we hear our doctors move quickly into prescribing medicine, as though this is all they know to do:

Doctor: (formally and with no affect) Well, Ms. Carson, let's see what medication we can start giving you to help you sleep better.

Though the doctor in these examples is doing his job and trying to be efficient, these responses are a total discounting of the patient's entire communication about her fears and despair. They lack both Warmth *and* Empathy. The doctor is letting her know in no uncertain terms that it's inappropriate for her to bring her emotional issues to him. Yet, we all know now that the physical/emotional connection in the disease process is profoundly interwoven. Though most physicians do not have time to "be therapists" or go into heavy emotional process with their patients, there are always quick, therapeutic responses that allow the patient to feel better, rather than feeling shut down or embarrassed, both of which are anti-therapeutic.

Physical healing is rarely permanent unless we have healed at the level of heart and soul. In severe emotional crises, sometimes the best therapeutic strategy is to help the patient work on through the feelings, similar to helping a patient to die with dignity.

Dr. Jim reminds us that on a busy day, you can add a few minutes of more focused time to one patient and subtract a bit of time from another patient who is at the office for a routine visit. And when time is really tight, acknowledging the patient and scheduling a visit with more time can validate the patient's needs in a way they will appreciate.

Heart feeling is the very opposite of cool, removed rationality. The heart unites us while the intellect divides us. When we drop the mask of separateness and speak to another person "heart to heart," our common bond overrides any sense of separateness. It links us as fellow travelers on this human journey fraught with both sorrow and joy. The bridge of the heart allows genuine dialogue to take place and grounds us in the absolute truth of the moment.

When your heart is open, you will respond just naturally to another's pain with Empathy and Warmth. You can actually experience both personal compassion and impersonal objectivity simultaneously with an open heart. And by the way, we are not the only species who suffers. Every species in creation has pain. But suffering is holding onto pain and contains a mental component of catastrophic thinking. If you can help your patients let go of catastrophic thinking, by calm empathetic connection, you've gone a long way toward helping them avoid creating more illness. *Thought is creative!* And we must never forget that.

An atmosphere of unconditional love encourages healing and well-being of both the helper and the one receiving the help. Through open-heart sharing with one's doctor, the patient will experience a peaceful feeling of warm release right in the center of his or her chest.

A heart that is emotionally constricted or contracted is full of unexpressed sorrow or even anger, and often can also be filled with piles of resentment that have never been released. It will eat up your precious energy to live with a closed heart. These pent-up feelings will turn to depression at some point if you never allow them to express, and can even make you sick. When you see a patient you feel is blocked emotionally to the detriment of his or her physical well-being, you can have places to refer the patient to that focuses on emotional healing. Your recommendation can open a door for these types of patients that could save their lives.

The link between sensory pain and emotional suffering, we now know, is rooted in our nervous system, utilizing the same neurotransmitters, such as serotonin, and both are processed in the same place in the brain. If an emotional problem persists for a long period of time, the brain's distress signals stay switched on, causing us to continue reacting in the same dysfunctional manner to the point that even the muscles can get sore and symptoms of fibromyalgia can occur (8).

## And Here Are Some Traps:

Becoming overly involved with patients and creating an emotional dependency is a way of getting stuck in Warmth—when too much closeness or personal need is evident on either side of the relationship.

Another trap is the other extreme of maintaining excessive emotional distance and reserve, believing that you are "being professional." You can remain professional, but caring by maintaining the balance between mind and heart advocated here.

### *Self-reflection:*

Recently, a friend of mine was commenting on having seen a doctor crying with a family he had just had to inform of the death of their child. He held the mother in his arms, with tears running down his face. And this occurred on the same day she had also watched another doctor tell a family their son would never walk again, then abruptly turn and walk out of the room with no more conversation about it. These are both extremes, of course. . . but worth pondering. Where do you just naturally fit along this continuum?

People incapable of Warmth have usually been raised in a family that had extreme and rigid family rules, devoid of unconditional love. For example, a family might be heavily into society and the formality of stately, reserved language and body movements that often accompany this aristocratic lifestyle. Or, some families have a background of addiction, which usually distorts emotional honesty in a family. At Dr. Jim's medical school, 40% of the med students identified themselves as coming from a family with an addiction problem. If so, you may be limiting your humanness in this very human, sensual world. And what a shame that is!

What might it be that causes you to feel too vulnerable to use more Warmth with your patients? What message do you tell yourself about this? Usually, you'll say it's too dangerous. As mentioned earlier, we can mistake being heartfelt as being too emotional, too feminine, or just plain weak. Sometimes people even believe that allowing conscious feeling of these emotions is a complete waste of time. Yet, the research today is clearly revealing the crucial importance of the relationship between mind, emotional happiness, and body—even recently making the cover of both *Newsweek* and *Time* magazines (7). We simply cannot ignore this fact!

The heart is a level of consciousness, or state of being, beyond ego needs. We drop defensiveness, our need to be right, or any kind of selfish needs and just listen and respond with total presence and concern. Coming from the heart has nothing to do with passion or sentimentality or excessive emotionalism. What we feel in our hearts will always be telling us exactly what's going on in any current situation, regardless of what our intellects may be trying to convince us of. The heart is reality. It cannot lie; it can only speak or feel the unadulterated truth.

When we are emotionally clear, we can trust our feelings. To withhold yourself from being openhearted in life means you have to create a subpersonality that is artificial, rigid, cold, detached, or simply out of touch with what's really going on in the moment. You may have developed a subpersonality that's always in need of being in total control. If so, you may have buried yourself in your intellect, finding constant ways to disengage with others and remain aloof.

Sometimes you'll hear about someone: "He's so dense, he could walk in a room where two people are about to kill each other and not even notice." This is a person who is completely out of touch with the more soulful, intuitive side of life. And what a limited way to live.

Perhaps it's time for you to re-examine your way of being if you see that you are closed and too detached in your communication with others. See what you can do about opening your heart. Little children are naturally outgoing and expressive of their feelings, until they are taught by rigid, uptight adults to repress their normal responses to life. So where do these feelings go? They become blocked anger, hurt, and grief, stuffed in the closets of our subconscious minds. And they will tend to burst out in rage or sexual or addictive acting-out if not consciously recognized and expressed. Or, conversely, these blocked emotions may just sit there, keeping you distant in all your relationships. You may be in need of much emotional healing yourself!

The emotional aspect of yourself does not heal by just thinking about your issues, however. Emotions function like water, and heal through the law of thermodynamics: Like carting around a full bucket of dirty water in your solar plexus and chest, pent-up emotions are heavy and must be emptied and "bled out" in order to heal. Talking about one's feelings can be an honest first step, but usually not enough for true relief. Certain experiential methods such as music therapy, the breathwork meditation technique available at the Eupsychia Institute healing programs, and other emotional release techniques in a safe, contained setting, are required to really heal our emotional bodies. If you tend to be an intellectual, your mind will need to give your heart permission to feel. Otherwise, you will continue to talk yourself out of opening your heart with the many unconscious rationalizations we intellectuals are so good at coming up with!

Take some time now, if you will, to just reflect on what "Warmth" really means in your personality structure. And see if you can allow this quality to blossom in your own natural way, both in your professional practice and certainly with your family and friends. If you are too cold and rigid in your response to others and to life, a transformation may be required. And I believe you're ready for this, or you wouldn't have read this far.

# CHAPTER FIVE

# Self-Disclosure

DEFINITION: The act of exposing one's own feeling, attitudes, beliefs, and experiences with another.

DESCRIPTION: This is the act of sharing the doctor's own feelings and life experiences with a patient for the sake of the patient. The research on Self-disclosure was mixed: it must be meaningful and relevant both in content and context to be therapeutic. It must be used with an accurate sense of timing and appropriateness, with a good idea of how the patient will make use of the information disclosed. It is never used for the doctor's own need to confess or vent.

I am a naturally self-disclosing therapist. But I learned years ago that disclosing too much about myself in the first few visits with my clients turned out to be a mistake. It is natural for new clients to need to see you as an "expert," someone well advanced over their own problematic ways. For you to start right out sharing too much about your own difficulties in life can discourage a patient from using you as a guide. Even though later on, it is healthy for the doctor/patient relationship to balance out more, at first, your patients need to see you in your strengths. Then, once rapport is well established, the two of you can become more equal and open with one another. So with this variable, watch out for timing.

**Self-Disclosure in action:**

Patient: (After being shown her medical tests that reveal she is suffering from fibromyalgia.) I feel so stupid. I've let myself be labeled a hypochondriac and an emotional basket case now for months, trying to find help with this awful way I've been feeling. No one would believe me, and everyone got sick of listening to me complain —to the point that I could no longer trust my own experience.

Doctor: I hope you won't be too hard on yourself about this. I've seen this sort of thing happen more often than you'd think. In fact, the very same thing happened to me a few years ago, when I lost all my energy and started complaining constantly. And, most of all, to my poor husband. I, too, started feeling like there was no medical reason for this, and thought I was just making it up. Then, finally, I went for tests and was diagnosed with extremely low thyroid.

Patient: Well, that sure does make me feel better. Thank you for telling me this.

Listening with interest to your patient's story and providing solace for her misery while she was seeking help may be the strongest medicine of all for this woman: a friendly doctor/ patient relationship. When she knows her doctor can be her friend, a trusting relationship ensues, where she feels valued and taken care of. Studies show that patients who have healthy relationships with their doctors who behave as friends get better clinical results.

In the above dialogue, Self-disclosure was appropriate and perfectly fitting for this patient's situation. Since patients often look up to their health care giver as someone more evolved than they are, to hear a professional confess a similar failing is a highly therapeutic interchange, one that brings a strong sense of "I'm okay" and relief to the patient. She knows she can communicate freely with this doctor and feel understood.

What some physicians may not realize is their patient may have had an non-caring, unresponsive mother or father, and may be starved for recognition and nurturing from an authority figure. Physicians are indeed authority figures. And it is true that some people go from doctor to doctor, seeking that intimate, nurturing support they have failed to get all their lives. There are limits, of course, to what a doctor can do for a needy patient like this, but Self-disclosure used appropriately can be a way to ease the over-under doctor/patient relationship that can lift the patient's self esteem.

Another form of Self-disclosure-in-action can include Empathy: "I know how you feel. I've 'been there' with this same kind of situation in my own family." (And you don't always need to give the details.) Or, Genuineness and a self-disclosing statement will make excellent helpmates: "Hearing you say this brings up the feelings I had back before I was diagnosed with low thyroid and thought I'd become a hypochondriac."

Sometimes a patient will even ask a health care professional outright if they've ever had such an experience. They are seeking more of a personal connection with their care giver, but not inappropriately. Following are some toxic responses in this instance:

**Toxic Responses:**

Doctor: "My personal life really isn't any of your concern. Let's get back to business here."

Even though this doctor may not be comfortable talking about herself, there are several ways she could have answered that question without putting down the patient. She could have said, "Look, our time is so short, let's focus on you so we can give you as much as possible today."

Here's another type of toxic response:

Doctor: "Yes, I've had this same problem. Years ago I developed low thyroid and it was a time in my life when our children were young and my husband was jobless and so much depended on me. It all even led to my husband and me having a serious problem in our marriage. . ." (Then the doctor continues to vent for 5 or so minutes of this patient's time).

This has become a monologue where the doctor has lost touch with why she is even sharing this information with her patient. She's gotten lost in her own story. The emphasis is no longer on the patient but has switched to the doctor, almost like a role reversal. This is a misuse of Self-disclosure.

Here's another example of a misuse of Self-disclosure:

Patient: (a young woman 19 years old, getting a physical examination before her upcoming marriage) I've not ever slept with my fiancée. My family is very religious and believes premarital sex is a sin. What do you think about this?

Doctor: "Well, I think it's best to know your partner sexually before you marry him. What if you two are completely incompatible? I don't confuse religion with issues around my sex life, and this saved me once from a terrible mistake."

The doctor is projecting her own values on the patient. And since this young woman is no doubt looking up to her doctor as an expert, she is being encouraged to just blindly transgress the values under which she was raised. Both the doctor and patient live in a sex-saturated culture and this young woman has maintained her values until this point, showing her serious commitment to abstinence. For her to now rush out and have sex with her fiancée could bring about serious guilt issues, or even a family crisis. Much deeper exploration of this issue is warranted. This is a thoughtless form of Self-disclosure.

### *Self-reflection:*

How comfortable are you about talking about yourself and your own life experiences? Perhaps you came from a family where it wasn't safe to share much about your own feelings and beliefs, and you just learned to keep away from any forms of Self-disclosure.

Or, the opposite can be true: That you talk too much, and can literally get carried away talking about yourself. I was with a physician recently, who went on and on about his miserable relationship with his wife during my office visit. His wife even called him on his cell phone during my time with him, and they proceeded to argue in front of me. Then, after hanging up, he processed more with me. I left that day feeling like he owed *me* a fee!

Your own personal style of communicating may fall into either of these more extreme categories, or you may see that you already use Self-disclosure quite naturally and appropriately. Getting feedback from a spouse or close friend about this might be wise. We often don't realize how we come across when communicating with others.

I recall a very poignant piece of feedback I received from a close friend once as I was going on and on about something—when she had actually come to me for help that day. She said, very lovingly, "Now, this is the fifth time you're going to tell me this. But if you really need to tell it again, I will really listen." This was one of the most therapeutic responses I've ever received from anyone. I didn't even feel judged, just amused at my lack of consciousness. We had a good laugh. The gentle confrontation taught me to take note of how I can sometimes become too self-preoccupied, forgetting the context for the disclosure.

## Conclusion

The personality variables you've studied thus far have all been rapport-building, supportive communication skills. Rapport-building conversations will always have an accepting, respectful, warm, and comprehending tone. And again, you already possess these traits; you just need to remember to use them when they are needed. They are designed to aid your patients in feeling safe and supportive in both their emotional and physical process of seeking health and healing, or of facing reality. When rapport is established, your patient feels that you care. Dr Jim regularly uses Self-disclosure to decrease patient resistance to therapeutic suggestions.

During the first few office visits with a patient, these rapport-building traits are essential. The more challenging ones that follow must be saved until you sense a therapeutic bond has been developed with a patient.

The next three qualities we'll study are the more assertive or exacting aspects of dialogue, where therapeutic confrontation or boundary setting of some kind may be required.

However, it's crucial that you always remember that *support must precede challenge* for these more confrontational interchanges to be taken seriously or effectively by your patient. This is a cardinal rule in therapeutic relating. It's been found that confronting a client before rapport is established simply does not work. The patient will find a way to either disregard your confrontation, or will become angry or argumentative with you, and seek another physician. If there is no rapport established, your patient doesn't trust that you care enough to listen to you when you challenge them. They can walk away saying to themselves, "What does she know? She has no idea what I'm really going through." Or, it can also be taken as "Why should I listen to her? She lives in a whole different world than I do." So the confrontation can be easily dismissed as unkind or irrelevant.

Research in the field of counseling and psychotherapy has shown that peer feedback is usually more effective than feedback from an expert for these reasons: It's easy to dismiss an expert you can't relate to. Yet, when peers start giving you the same message about how you need to change, you can relate to them as friends who really know you, or as associates who live on your same level in life. That "expert" who is giving you this advice doesn't really know you that well, and may just be doing his or her job.

When rapport is established with your patients, they know that you care. And you will sense this in the way they relate to you. Also, they have heard enough of your humanness by now to know you have been through similar challenges in your own life and really do understand. Your confrontation of them will seem like real caring and concern rather than hurtful feedback.

Following are the three personality variables, Concreteness, Immediacy, and Confrontation, we use when needing to directly accost someone seeking our aid with a reality they may be having a hard time facing. You may find these traits harder or easier for you than the rapport-building ones, depending on your natural way of being.

## Chapter Six

# Concreteness

DEFINITION: This is the act of getting to the real specific details of relevant concerns—keeping your communication focused and to the point.

DESCRIPTION: Characterized by statements concerning the immediate experience of specific realities, this trait is never abstract, general, or idealistic in its expression. It is always personal, and right to the point.

Concreteness keeps you and the patient from going off on tangents or getting into generalizations or abstract discussions with your patients that lead nowhere.

This quality helps you remember to notice your patients' unique ways of avoiding their reality by artfully drawing them back to the issues at hand that are not being dealt with in a health-producing manner. It also helps you stay on the mark—especially in this current world of managed care, when your time is extremely short with each patient. Because of such time constraints, combined with some of the supportive variables already discussed, Concreteness is a valuable tool for most physicians to master.

**Concreteness-in-action:**

> Patient: Well, I know lots of people have the kind of leukemia I have. Some survive. Others don't. I just heard on the news yesterday. . . .

> Doctor: (gently interrupts, warm voice) Loretta, statistics and general information about your disease can be helpful for you to know. But I'd rather hear how *you* are feeling. . . how *you* are doing with this disease process you're currently living with. I want to hear what symptoms you're still having, how the new medicine is working. . . . Let's talk about you.

We often want to avoid how we are feeling about some painful issue by escaping into generalities that are much safer to focus on than the intimate personal feelings we might be having about a devastating illness. Here, the doctor has pulled her back to her own experience and saved time for the therapeutic portion of the office call. Now this session can be more productive.

We never grow much from hearing about other people "in general." In fact, when we're hurting or fearful about something happening in our lives, it always seems like we are unique in that situation. So another type of concrete response could be commenting on the process rather than the content of the patient's statement. This type of therapeutic response includes high levels of Empathy as well. Here's an example:

> Doctor: I realize this is so affecting you, really, in every area of your life. So how are you doing with all this right now? Perhaps I can offer some resources for you if I know more about what you might be needing.

Patients and clients can be quite uncomfortable at the first part of a session with us. General and superficial conversation is a way to avoid deeper feelings. This response above is helpful because it not only cuts to the chase, but also adds an offer of help and hope.

Years ago I learned from one of my mentors how to very quickly help my clients get to the core issue they are needing to address. It was by using one simple question over and over several times! The question is, "Can you be more specific?"

This is a classic way of using Concreteness. And I've found to my surprise that every time I say this back to my clients, they go deeper into their feelings, closer to the true source of the real difficulty, until finally they will just burst out with the bottom-line issue that's really bothering them. Here's an example of what I mean:

Client: I just hate living here. I feel bad so much of the time. I think I need to move.

Counselor: Can you be more specific?

Client: I can't stand how it feels living in my house.

Counselor: Can you be *more* specific?

Client: I used to love it, but now there are so many things I can't stand about it anymore.

Counselor: What things are you talking about specifically? What's wrong with your house?

Client: (yells with much emotion) If my sister doesn't leave,

I'm going to go crazy! I can't stand her living with us!

Now we're there. This is the issue.

You can adapt this type of questioning to your times with your patients when you feel they are all over the place in speaking with you about their health issues. It's so simple, yet extremely effective.

**Toxic Responses:**

Doctor: Let's get to the point here. We don't have time to explore the research or public opinion. We are already running late. I have another appointment in five minutes.

Concreteness must never sound rude—never with a curt or dismissive tone. This can cause the patient to feel attacked in the hands of an arrogant or aloof provider she must be counting on for her physical health. Concreteness must be coupled with the qualities of Warmth and a great deal of Respect to be a useful communication skill.

In the above example, the doctor is reminding his patient that he isn't really as important as the next appointment he mustn't be late for. Though everything he says is true, the response is too curt.

Another form of toxic response is when a physician enters into a long, unhelpful dialogue about the disease in general, using medical jargon and scientific research findings the patient cannot even comprehend. Jargon in any profession is a conversation stopper, as it can make our clients feel dumb or uneducated. We need to remember to speak on their level as much as possible.

Sometimes, even when you do use Concreteness to bring patients back to their reality, they will continue to use gossip and generalizations to avoid their feelings. If they are not ready to work on issues of fear or self-doubt connected with a disease process, this need for avoidance can be respected with a comment such as:

"I can tell you're just needing some time to think about all this, or to feel it through. It may be just too scary to face all at once. We can talk about it later, but we do have to deal with this situation on several levels for you to receive the help you need. So let me know when you're ready."

Here, the doctor is being realistic, keeping to the point, and also letting the patient know he's there for her whenever she's ready to deal with her diagnosis directly. Within reason, it's best the doctor not jump too far ahead of where the patient is in dealing with a critical diagnosis.

Dr. Jim reminds us that the "one step at a time" approach used in addiction recovery is a very effective model for realistically going through the necessary states of change. Instead of solely advocating the eventual goal of abstinence, the provider moves the patient one step at a time at each contact. Gradually the patient is guided from pre-contemplation to contemplation, then to readiness, and later to action, and finally to maintenance of abstinence.

High-functioning psychotherapists know how to stay with their clients right where they're at. Yet, in certain severe medical issues, time may be of the essence, and wasting time could even be life threatening. So the use of this personality trait is an important one for physicians to develop therapeutically.

## And Here's A Trap:

Research shows most providers interrupt the patient's story before the end of the first minute of the interview. This is over-applying Concreteness, as multiple open-ended questions allow a broader net for obtaining information and will clearly demonstrate to one's patients that they are being heard.

You can learn to let the patient tell her story before using Concreteness to clarify the important details. This will help build the rapport needed before any more confrontive dialogue might need to take place.

### Self-reflection:

You might want to reflect on your style of communicating, asking yourself what kind of feedback have you been given fairly consistently in your life about how you come across. Are you felt to be naturally friendly and rather talkative, or are you seen as more aloof and non-disclosing, keeping your personal thoughts "close to your chest."

If you're the more reserved type, you will be better at Concreteness than some of us are. I am a talker! So when tested in this research, I functioned very low on the use of this personality variable, which didn't come naturally for me at all. I had to practice it over and over to gain the confidence and the skill involved. I found that I was uncomfortable with silence and often used words to comfort myself when my client would stop talking. With practice, I've learned to actually enjoy silence, and even use it as a therapeutic tool.

How about you? Do you just naturally tend to talk too much, veering off the subject a lot, in making conversation? If so, this might mean you are also uncomfortable being in the here and now with your patients, especially when their issues are scary or painful.

Making conscious the need for Concreteness with patients will vividly bring to your awareness the times when it's absent. You will start to notice you are wasting precious time in irrelevant talk and can immediately start to implement your inherent quality of being concrete.

70

## Chapter Seven

# Immediacy

DEFINITION: Stated self-evident, direct awareness in the
present moment

DESCRIPTION: This conversational trait deals with the feelings between the doctor and the patient in the here and
now. It points out in open sharing what is going on
between the two of you in the moment, taking the emphasis off the content of the patient's problems and plac-
ing it on the actual process going on between the two of
you right now.

Immediacy is the most "dangerous" of all the traits to use—
and therefore, usually the most avoided! It will remove all defenses occurring between the two of you and bring issues to the
surface you may find uncomfortable to deal with, right here
and now. When you ask your patient, "What's going on with
you right now in relation to me?" you may not get the answer
you'd like to hear. And once shared, a confrontation may occur.

However, the research indicates that this is one of the most
useful, effective therapeutic variables for rapid movement beyond stiff, stuck, or dead feelings occurring between the caregiver
and the patient. Immediacy helps us cut to the chase when there

is an obvious dynamic going on between the two of you that needs addressing.

## Immediacy-in-action:
(when what's happening in the moment feels negative)

> Doctor: Marty, it feels like you are angry with me right now. And, golly, if I'm right, I'd sure like to clear this up really fast so we can proceed with your plans for treatment. Are you mad at me?

> Marty: Well, no. . . . I mean, yes. Oh, maybe a little. . . . Shoot! I don't know. . . .

> Doctor: Come on now. . . . Tell me what's bothering you. (gently, with a little humor in his tone) I can take it.

> Marty: Well, you seem more distracted and in a hurry than usual. So yes, I'm upset. I'm anxious about all this medical information I'm getting, and I really need to talk about it. But I feel like I'm intruding on your time.

> Doctor: (pauses. . . then leans forward with a warm, conversational tone) You know, you're right. I am more hurried and more stressed today. We had an emergency this morning that's put me way off schedule. I'm sorry that this is showing so much in my behavior. Let's start over, and I do want to give you the time you need this morning. My next patient can just wait a little longer.

You'll notice a combination of Self-disclosure, Immediacy,

and Warmth is all at play here. And all are useful to help this patient feel heard and better about her very appropriate needs. After all, her doctor may be the only resource she has for the questions concerning her.

It is so often true that physicians feel pressed for time. And patients today are more demanding of a therapeutic relationship with their doctors than in the past. They want more dialogue, more give-and-take, more medical or alternative options discussed in an intelligent, respectful manner. They often ask for more emotional support as well. And this is all happening at a time when insurance companies and managed care are demanding that doctors increase their patient-load, which means requiring them to spend less time with each patient.

It's perfectly all right for you to share with your patients your own frustration about this lack of time problem that exists in your practice. With heartfelt Self-disclosure and a willingness to use this quality of Immediacy, you can go a long way toward developing a very understanding and manageable experience in the short time you have with each patient. These matters just need to be brought to the table and discussed openly, not buried underneath layers of repressed disappointment or hostility.

Here's another way this skill can sound:

Doctor: I'm aware you are fidgeting in your chair and looking out the window as I'm telling you this, Marty. Can you tell me what's going on? How are you relating to what I'm saying right now?

Patient: I'm nervous, that's all. This is really hard for me. And I guess it's hard for me to tell you I want to go for a second opinion. It doesn't mean I don't trust you, it's just that this is so serious, and I'm really scared. . . . And,

I don't want to hurt your feelings.

The doctor is pointing out to this patient what he is observing in her behavior. This usually elicits immediacy quite naturally between the two of you. And it brought up the real issue going on between them.

**Immediacy-in-action:**
(when the feelings of the moment are positive between a male doctor and his female patient)

Patient: I've brought you this little gift today. It's not much, but I wanted you to have it. It's just a token that means something special to me. I'm just so grateful for all you've done for me. I'm feeling really close to you right now.

Doctor: Well, thanks, Marty. This is very kind of you. I appreciate your willingness to tell me this. I know you've been through the ringer lately. And I realize I don't have much time with you, but I do care deeply about what you and your family are going through and I'm willing to help all I can as your physician.

Here, it's important that the doctor not give any mixed messages that could open the door for romantic or too intimate feelings from this patient. In the statement above, the doctor remains clean and clear about his professional role with this patient and the reality of the time they share as doctor/patient. Yet, he's not holding back from being warm, sensitive, and respectful of her feelings. This is a clear example of how to deal with any potential transference issues, as discussed earlier.

**Toxic Responses:**

Most toxic responses, when Immediacy is called for, will contain this quality's opposites: being too superficial, too discounting, or too oblivious of what's going on in the room at the moment.

When a patient offers you some gift or act of kindness and appreciation, it's important that you respond in a kind manner, even though you may need to draw a boundary around the relationship, to keep it professional. A toxic response would be insulting or too non-caring, such as:

Doctor: Sorry, Marty, I don't take gifts from my patients. Now, let's get down to business here. I need to go over these test results with you.

This is too cold and abrupt. If you don't take gifts, there's a nicer way of saying this, such as "Well, thanks so much, Marty. I appreciate your kindness. However, I decided a long time ago not to accept gifts from my patients. It's just a policy I try to uphold. I hope you understand."

Now here's a very toxic, dangerous response:

Marty: I've brought you a little gift today. It's not much, but I just wanted to give you something because I'm feeling so grateful to you and so close to you right now. (adoringly) You've just about saved my life.

Doctor: Thanks, Mary. I feel close to you as well. I will cherish this beautiful book mark, and will think of you every time I use it. Thanks so much.

This type of response lacks the necessary boundary that must remain intact between a physician and one's patients. She could misinterpret this as a personal, or even romantic or sexual response—especially if she is needy in this area of her life. As mentioned earlier, it's very easy for patients to have romantic crushes on their doctors and too much warmth and friendliness can feed their fantasies that the doctor is responding romantically.

## A Note about Seduction: Using Immediacy to combat transference issues with a patient

If a patient "comes on to you" in a seductive manner, eliciting a romantic or sexual response from you, Immediacy can be a valuable resource in your conversations with this patient. You can ask directly what the patient is feeling toward you, and offer responses that have no ambiguity about your refusal to go there. And in the now, you can do this in a way that doesn't insult the patient. You can use comments that honor her feelings and point her toward finding this kind of love in her life with someone appropriate, while letting her know under no uncertain terms that you are not available.

You might want to re-read the section on Transference/ Counter-transference in Chapter Two.

Never be naïve about how your patients, especially lonely ones who use seduction as a way of being noticed, fall so easily into the dynamics of transference. Be constantly on your guard—especially if you are a naturally friendly, easy to be with, person. A needy woman, for example, might even seek out an attractive male doctor, hoping to get some badly needed personal attention. I've had cases where the woman was convinced her doctor was in love with her by the look in his eye.

Therapists, physicians, and ministers have to deal with transference and counter-transference issues all the time because it's so easy to misinterpret therapeutic helping with romantic intimacy. Here's a reminder: "Transference" means the patient's way of confusing you with a lover or a parent. And "counter-transference" is when the helper has romantic/sexual stirrings toward the one seeking help.

**Here Are Some More Traps:**

Avoiding acknowledgment of the emotional issues your patient is experiencing, fearfully hoping a touchy problem like the patient's self-destructive risk-taking behavior will just go away.

Cutting off abruptly when feeling the patient is not responding—subtly, but angrily pushing the patient back. I've heard therapists tell me "the client is not ready for therapy" when, in fact, the therapist wasn't being effective! We must all be careful to not blame our clients when we feel they are being noncompliant until we've examined our own effectiveness and willingness to look at our own part in this failure.

Feeding into the patient's dysfunction to satisfy personal ego needs, by playing the flirtation game. Much is already being said here about transference and counter-transference.

*Self-reflection:*

So often physicians are faced with their patients' deepest emotional reactions to hearing they have a serious, perhaps even life-threatening illness. And remember, an emotionally healing relationship between you and your patients plays a vital role in their medical care.

In Advances, the *Journal of Mind-Body Health*, their Winter, 1997 issue focused on the role of Self in healthy cancer survivorship. Dr. Keith I. Block's research (quoted on page 6), from The Cancer Institute at Edgewater Medical Center in Chicago, found that when faced with the threat of cancer, depending on its severity, the emotional tenor of one's reaction can range from reasonable concern to downright overwhelming panic. Coping responses such as despair and helplessness were found to trigger a cascade of neuroendocrine processes that compromise the very immune mechanisms needed to keep malignant tumors and micrometastases at bay. And positive coping behaviors appeared to help keep the immune system actively engaged in neoplastic surveillance and cytotoxic activities, which discouraged the progression of the cancer.

I cannot stress strongly enough the need for emotional healing to accompany physical treatment in one's illness process. Since the use of Immediacy can bring up all sorts of emotionally intimate issues with your patients, you might ask yourself,

> "What issues come up for me when I'm called upon to bring up these very personal feelings in my conversations with my patients?"

> "How comfortable am I with the confrontations in the moment that arise from using this therapeutic tool?"

> "Do I hide behind my professionalism? If so, what am I hiding from? What is it that I fear?"

An honest evaluation of these questions will help you uncover any unhealed issues of your own that might hinder your most effective, healthy way of being with your patients. Finding the therapeutic balance between "professionalism" and "personal relating" is essential in your life with your patients, because it's been found that regardless of the diagnosis, a patient whose doctor is a good-hearted friend won't ever need to worry about being abandoned, scolded, or uncared for. The relationship itself is the safe and reliable emotional container and elicits a sense of well-being in one's patients. Yet, building a healthy relationship takes time—something managed care has conspired to remove from most health care givers. I know of some doctors who are now refusing to take insurance so they can avoid the managed care process and relate to their patients more in the old-fashioned way of the country doc who really cared!

Our current health care system works against the opportunity for much therapeutic relating between doctors and their patients. So you have to be creative and find ways for this to happen in the shortest amounts of time. Medical schools at Harvard, Columbia, Duke, and the University of Arizona are creating programs helping physicians to stop focusing exclusively on disease, toward promoting the doctor/patient relationship, wellness and prevention. And all this must be done realizing the danger of transference and seductive/sexual issues arising in some needy patients.

More and more, with the paradigm shifts occurring now in our medical world, you must be clear and healthy in terms of meeting your own emotional and sexual needs so as not to ever be susceptible to any form of dysfunctional relating with a needy, frightened, lonely, or seductive patient. Yet, at the same time, you are required to respect the fact that emotional healing is essential for physical well-being, and the doctor/patient relationship is being shown more and more to be of extreme importance in this regard. The relationship itself *should* provide a safety net for anything that might hinder your patients' well-being. And if it's not, what might be missing in the necessary therapeutic attitude required of you for your patients' health?

Reflect on these paradigm shifts attempting to emerge in your field, and ask yourself how you feel about changes you may need to make within yourself. Being the "outside expert" in the life of another is beginning to show cracks in its armor. Patients today are venturing away from unfriendly conventional medical practitioners, now studying and in search of less technical healing practices that keep the human factor as a priority. Many today are seeing that dispensing pills and rigid medical procedures for everything is an incomplete and often unsatisfactory model of health care.

Are you willing to undergo whatever shift in consciousness you may need to make in order to be in closer affiliation with the times? In today's climate, doctors and patients alike can become allies in seeking ways to sustain hope and discover the meaning in suffering together. As quoted in *Newsweek*'s issue on *The New Science of Mind & Body*: "The value of the doctor-patient relationship is not always easy to measure, but it is always immeasurable" (9).

Patients today expect their doctors to remember their name!

CHAPTER EIGHT

# Confrontation

DEFINITION: To compel another to face, and take responsibility for, some dangerous, disturbing, or untruthful communication or situation being observed.

DESCRIPTION: This is the act of bringing the patient face to face with his or her reality, as you perceive it. There will be two types of confrontation most often required in the medical profession:

1) when the patient is resisting, or not following a prescribed treatment plan; and

2) when the patient and family members are in denial about one's illness and neglecting to take needed actions.

Confrontation will often precipitate a crisis in any relationship. It can be therapeutic or it can be toxic, depending on how it's stated and the energy behind it. If done therapeutically, a confrontation can bring about a breakthrough in your patient's life.

Therapeutic confrontation is a most crucial communication skill when dealing with patients who tend to go into unconscious denial or rationalizations, or in any way have trouble accepting or taking responsibility for what's at hand. Serious and life-threatening illnesses can certainly cause such unconscious denial to happen in patients and in their family members as well.

Often, the worse the sickness, the more necessary will become the need to confront for the sake of the patient's well-being. We needn't think of confrontation as being negative just because it's confrontive; it can really be a healer. Some are even confrontations to increase in an area of personal strength, such as: "I hear you putting yourself down right now, yet I've seen you be very productive in this area of your life. You have a real talent for this I don't see you owning."

Regardless of the content of what we need to confront, we must take responsibility for how we meet our patients head-on. When a discrepancy occurs, we want to know how to do it therapeutically rather than "hitting below the belt."

Healthy confrontation comes from a clear mind and heart, from someone with no ax to grind but who just sees that the patient needs to face a denied reality. The doctor confronts for the sake of the patient's well-being, not to meet some psychological need of her own. And remember, rapport must already be established before you can expect a confrontation to take hold.

No one likes to be reminded of things they would prefer to avoid seeing or dealing with, especially when they concern serious health issues. This is why our psyches create unconscious denial mechanisms that hold us away from uncomfortable truths. So often, it will be up to you to cut through denial and bring the reality to the forefront. This may even need to be done over and over during your patient's healing or dying process.

So how do you learn to say things that are confrontational but essential to your patient's well-being in a way that is therapeutic? Here are some examples that might be useful:

## Therapeutic Confrontation-in-action:

Doctor: John, I'm noticing your speech is slurred today and your thinking seems vague and unclear. I'm really concerned. So tell me the truth now: Are you tampering with your seizure medication dosages again?

John: (hesitantly) Well. . . no, not really too much. I'm just not happy with how I've been feeling lately. So I did slow down on the evening dose. You know I don't do well on any kind of strong medicine. And my herbalist friend says I need to try some of her supplements instead. So I am a bit confused right now.

Doctor: Please, John, just tell me what you're taking, or not taking. I need to know. You could be getting in real trouble here.

John: Well, yes. I s'pose so. My symptoms have increased, but not too bad. I'm just hazy and not knowing what to do. . . you know.

Doctor: I disagree that they are "not too bad." These symptoms are re-appearing again too often. And these are blackouts, remember? And they can happen anytime, and put you and others in serious danger. (notices John is looking out the window) John, I need you to focus with me here. Okay? (warm tone, but very sincere and engaged. Moves closer to his patient.) So help me out now. You and I both know this isn't working. What can we do with your medication that we can both feel good about? I need your advice *and* your cooperation. So let's start with what you've actually been taking. . . .

The doctor is showing his sincere concern, and is soliciting the participation of the patient in a respectful manner. Yet, he is sticking to his firmly held conviction that John needs his prescribed medication. This is highly therapeutic and will no doubt lead to the patient's desire to cooperate rather than argue or resist.

Obviously, there is rapport here. And the doctor has had experience with John already where this problem has needed confronting. Inviting the patient to be involved in the decision about his medication is an effective choice.

Situations such as this require more dialogue than a mere "stop it and listen to me" attitude, which would be a toxic way of handling this patient. When you know you must confront a patient, it's a good idea to reserve a few more minutes than your ordinary appointment time.

Here's another example of how therapeutic Confrontation sounds:

Doctor: Hi, Josie, how have you been doing since I last saw you? Tell me what's been going on.

Patient: Oh, I'm just fine. Things are good. How are you doing?

Doctor: Whoa, Josie! Something seems off here, woman. I look at you and see a loss of weight you couldn't afford to lose. You are pale and appear to even have the nervous jitters. And you're avoiding looking at me right now. Come on. . . . I'm on your side, remember? So tell me now, how are you *really* doing?

Here the doctor is seeing a discrepancy in what the patient is saying and the way she looks. Observing behaviors and appearance in the moment when contradictory with what the patient is saying is an efficient and forthright way to confront. Pointing out this discrepancy to the patient is a therapeutic response for several reasons: The doctor is noticing her, which always makes a patient feel attended to. There is an Immediacy proposition put into play, where the patient is called upon to notice she's not making eye contact or speaking her truth. And the doctor is using Warmth to remind her she's her friend and Josie is safe to speak her truth there with her physician.

**Toxic Responses:**

There are four ways confrontation becomes toxic:

1) Statements that induce guilt or that shame your patients are not only unhelpful, they exacerbate negative self-feelings and poor emotional health.

2) Anything sounding accusatory will produce a defensive reaction.

3) Preaching to your patients seldom works, either. No one likes to be "preached at," probably not even you.

4) And finally, if you have built up anger toward your patient, there will be too much energy in your confrontation. It will be "loaded" with your own unexpressed emotional issues, so that you will project these onto your patient

with more intensity than needed. For example, some of us have an over-investment in being right or being "minded." So when a patient ignores our assignments or our way of seeing something, we get bent out of shape and can even feel attacked. Or, we become authoritarian and speak to the patient as though she is a naughty child. And this lacks the quality of Respect.

Negative confrontations often begin with the word, "You." "You haven't. . ." "You are being. . . ." And "you statements" like this will nearly always sound accusatory or judgmental. Using "I" language is more helpful: "I am very concerned that you. . . ." "I'm at a loss here because I sense what's happening is. . . ." Using "I" language gives the recipient a chance to accept what's being said as *your* process and it doesn't push their defense buttons nearly so much. Then they're more likely to listen rather than react to what's being said. For example, in response to the above-mentioned case, here's how a toxic response might sound:

Doctor: You don't listen to me. I've told you this is the dosage you're to take. So that's it. If you can't follow my instructions, then I can't work with you. Here's another prescription for what I say you need. I can't do any more for you now. So if you'll excuse me, we're out of time.

This response completely discounts the patient's experience of being sensitive to his medication and his confusion about what is working and what isn't. It is an especially poor choice as pharmo-kinetics is showing wide variation in effective doses of many medicines. In this example, there is no dialogue about what's really the issue here. It contains no Empathy, Warmth or interest in the patient's issues, which is a lack of Respect. If you don't really know, or even care, what's going on with your patients, you can't expect to treat them holistically.

Or, sometimes a confrontation can sound too rude and accusatory, like this:

Patient: I just can't understand how that drug test turned positive. I've never in my life used that substance. This is a big mistake.

Doctor: Why aren't you being honest with me? I can tell you're lying.

Calling someone an outright liar is never helpful. . . even if the patient is obviously telling a lie. And arguing about whether or not the patient is lying is a waste of precious time. You can always therapeutically call a patient on his falsehoods by using Warmth, Immediacy, and therapeutic Confrontation—which would sound more like this:

"Gosh, Jim, I wish I could believe you. But I'm having a real problem doing it. The facts here are giving me a different story. Maybe you're afraid to tell me you've been using again? I'm really not about reporting you to anyone; I'm your doctor, not your judge."

Patients lie to their doctors usually for *three* reasons:

1) to please an authority figure

2) to keep from being reprimanded

3) to maintain an unacceptable behavior, such as an addiction or high risk sex practice

When you know your patient is lying and needs to be called on it, the best way to handle it is to tell her you are having trouble believing her because. . . and point out the discrepancy you are observing. There will always be a discrepancy between

1) what she's saying now and what she said or promised earlier;

2) what she's saying and how she looks or is behaving; or

3) what she says she's doing when you know that she's not doing it.

You can practice using "I" language when you observe discrepancies in a gentle but sincere tone, until this becomes second nature to you.

Timing is also important in utilizing Confrontation. If rapport has not been established, it's better to wait until it is. Just be a good listener and use a softer tone at first. Or, if your patient is too emotionally distraught to hear certain bad news or your disapproval of something, you might want to wait until she is calmer and more receptive. For physicians, however, because you sometimes deal with issues of life and death, you may not always be able to hold back on what needs an immediate confrontation. So you can always use Empathy, Genuineness, Warmth, and Self-disclosure to soften the blow and build up rapport.

## And Here's a Trap:

After becoming frustrated from failing multiple therapeutic approaches to a patient's denial, the practitioner may be tempted to simply drive the patient away through a rude or crude version of Confrontation. This can create an angry mindset of feeling betrayed in the noncompliant patient. This is not therapeutic. And it can become a seedbed for potential courtroom battles as well.

## *Self-reflection:*

Unlike psychotherapists, physicians do not have the time nor the expected responsibility to do deep, probing psychotherapy with their patients. However, it is important that you know how to deepen your patients into enough of their issues so that accurate medical decisions can be cooperatively made and followed. Sometimes, too, doctors need to make referrals to psychotherapists when they sense emotional blocks are in the way of the patient's treatment program. You need to know what resources you have for this type of service in your community.

Doctors are notoriously criticized for abruptly shutting the door on discussions with their patients, and often behaving as "the expert" with an arrogant attitude that the patient is not to question their authority. Confrontations with no Warmth or Empathy, or no willingness to even hear the patient's own viewpoint, can lead to much unnecessary resistance and denial in the patient.

Ask yourself whether or not you fall into this category of the "cold, aloof doctor with a superior attitude." And with extreme self-honesty, see what answer you come up with. If you have doubt, ask one or two of your best friends. Or perhaps even your spouse!

Therapeutic Confrontation often takes practice. None of us are very good with having to confront people. Even the word itself carries a negative connotation. But I must say, when my behavior or mind-set about something has caused me extreme difficulty in life, it's been these heartfelt confrontations by people who really care about me that have truly changed my life. I would even go further and say that some of my biggest adversaries have been my greatest teachers!

We must learn to not fear necessary confrontations. Instead, we can re-frame this unpopular word to mean "a loving way to help someone face the real truth about something important in their lives."

# Chapter Nine

# Potency

DEFINITION: This is the therapeutic variable in our personalities that wields the force of passion or authority that has the capacity to influence or affect thought or feeling.

DESCRIPTION: This variable is measuring the charismatic or magnetic quality of the helper. Potent therapists and physicians have presence. They are outgoing and expressive, and very obviously in command of themselves. They communicate a dynamic, involved attitude with their patients. They are carriers of hope and enthusiasm that "shows." Rating high in Potency allows your patients to have confidence in you as an effective doctor with life-giving qualities. They will believe in you and what you stand for, because you so obviously do.

People high in Potency often become popular leaders and guides for others. The potent physician would be able to bring out the vitality in his or her patients in ways that enhance the life force. And remember, it's the power of the life force itself that is always the healer of any ailment. Since it's known now that the doctor/patient relationship is, in itself, a therapeutic agent, it's obvious that Potency plays a major role in helping patients feel respected, valued, and cared for by their physician.

The research indicated that this personality trait cannot be taught, as can the eight traits we've already studied; one's potency is a matter of *being*; it's not about *doing*. Consequently, it will require conscious work on oneself—often by healing emotional issues stemming from your past. And sometimes this may require some counseling or other forms of psychotherapy or spiritual awakening programs that inspire personal transformation. I am definitely a resource for this type of program, if you are ever interested.

Potency is mainly your willingness to fully express yourself with openhearted dedication and zeal *vis a vis* others relating to you in life. There will be a relaxed confidence in one who is high in Potency. When they walk into a room, you can feel their presence. Potency cannot be "faked;" by its very nature, it is one's authenticity. It carries with it a strong statement of being completely at home with oneself.

The research underlying the material in this book found that potent therapists make the more effective therapists, because people really believe them, and view them as models of health and well-being.

Here is an example of how a potent physician sounds:

**Potency-in-action:**

Doctor: Hi there, William. (big smile) It's *really* good to see you. Man oh man! Are you looking great! I was so pleased to hear from your wife yesterday that you were feeling so much better. Your tests show there is no longer *any* sign of infection in your body now. Hooray! (reaches over, pats William on the knee). And congratulations, sir! Your wife said you've been impeccable in doing everything you were supposed to, and you really deserve the credit for conquering this one.

Here, the doctor willingly involves with this patient, and is coming out strongly with his own personality. This kind of positive expression from one's primary caregiver is "catching." It empowers the patient and enables him or her to feel that the doctor really cares.

Even for the natural introvert, this quality can be progressively developed. A medical setting is the doctor's 'environment,' and any practitioner can therefore constantly practice development of this trait. Put simply, Potency is simply believing in oneself and what one has to offer to the point that it shows. Some of the therapists who tested high in Potency were introverts. And their Potency came across more in a quiet confidence and a easy-going sense of humor about life.

**Toxic or Impotent Responses:**

Doctor: Good afternoon, Mr. Smith. (business-like manner) I have your latest test results here. You look clear of infection now (no affect). So we can make your next appointment for a month or two from now. Just see the receptionist as you leave.

This doctor is relating in a robot-like, overly professional manner, not encouraging any dialogue, nor is he giving the patient any "strokes" or even any notice for his effective healing process. He is holding himself away from involvement with this patient, and comes across as aloof. He is utilizing very little of his own inner power. He is not positively energizing the patient, or the encounter. Therefore, he won't be facilitating the release of any power in his patient.

People who score low in Potency are flat in affect, uninvolved and unexpressive. Therapists and physicians high in Potency know how to utilize their own inner power to bring forth more potency in those seeking their aid.

Giving patients positive feedback about their part in achieving a healthy recovery is always highly therapeutic; it encourages self-empowerment by activating the patient's desire to be creative and motivated to take charge of his own life. It helps them believe they have some power in life.

It the field of counseling and psychotherapy, it's been found that clients often leave sessions with counselors who lack Potency. Those we interviewed said they felt uninspired and certainly not helped. And some had even dropped out of therapy altogether, deciding psychotherapy is ineffective. There is little energy exchange between the helper and the client when this therapeutic variable is low or absent.

Here are some low-Potency responses:

Patient: I'm just so scared about all this, Dr. Matthews. I want to just double up my fists and yell at God! What on earth have I done to deserve this awful prognosis, when I've done everything to be healthy? Can you just tell me. . . ? (puts head in her hands)

Doctor: We needn't get into this today, Miss Carson. (little affect) We'll do our best to get you better. (behaving as though somewhat distracted) I'll see you again next week with a well-thought-out treatment plan. Here's another prescription for you in case you need it for pain.

Here, the doctor gets down to business in a professional manner.

There is certainly no complaint about that part. But what is missing here? He completely ignores the patient's affect and emotional cry for help, as though it is not worth listening to. His affect is way below that of his patient's, so she is not being met where she is living in her body at that moment in time. His way of responding to this patient will shut her down, whereas, if emotions are met with a similar level of response from the doctor, there can be an emotional release that's quite healing. And the doctor can proceed by offering compassion, with much Warmth, and Empathy.

**Here are Some Traps:**

You might use the excuse, "I'm just an introvert," rather than developing this empowered side of yourself for emotional balance and more enthusiasm in life. Perhaps you need more comfort with personal power used appropriately. Maybe in a family with siblings you were always the one who held yourself back.

The three shadow sides of Potency are:

1) arrogance — being too self-confident, to the point of feeling superior to others, and behaviors that appear to be ego-driven

If this is a danger for you, you may need a bit of humility training! And usually, the world will give this to you in ways you'll least expect.

2) superficiality — being excessively jovial and outgoing, used to avoid deep communication

When this is your issue, you might work on maintaining a real connection with patients. You can start out by going deeper with the patients you feel most at home with.

3) giving yourself away — using your energy to propel others who become dependent on your enthusiasm to feel a high.

There are "emotional vampires" out there who literally feed on our energy—and want to live vicariously through us. These types of people have boundary issues and like to get "high" on your enthusiasm about your life. When you don't meet their excessive emotional needs for intimacy and specialness, however, they often turn on you. This dynamic, in the medical model of therapy, is labeled "a borderline personality." And there is certainly some truth in this diagnostic label! Lots of times, these patients will go from doctor to doctor, looking for that one who will allow them to become completely enmeshed in their lives. When you sense this is the case, you'll know it by your own level of exhaustion, or sometimes even irritability. You'll need to use Immediacy and gentle Confrontation with this person to let them know you aren't willing—or even able—to do their emotional work for them. And you can empower them by stating your own belief in their capabilities.

It's important that you maintain professional boundaries with your patients and take care of your own personal needs to avoid vulnerability. Dr. Jim comments that as physcians there are some times when our natural potency is just not available. If some days we just don't have a lot to give because of a personal issue or possibly an " all nighter" in the ICU or the delivery room, we can validate the patient, and invite him or her back for another office call when we are more rested and have more time to spend with them.

## *Self-reflection:*

If you feel you are naturally high functioning in Potency, I hope this helps you feel validated in your remarkable ability to express your vivacious, enthusiastic or encouraging responses to your patients and to life in general.

If you feel you are low in this quality, perhaps you are shy. And if so, this just may be your natural way of being more comfortable—when not in the forefront. Or, you may be lacking in self-confidence for some reason. And if so, this would be causing you problems in other areas of your life as well, so it does need attention and perhaps some healing of old childhood issues. Or maybe you've just never thought about letting your enthusiasm for life show a bit more. Physicians no doubt have some of this trained out of them in medical school. But as we've said earlier, you can carry "being professional and emotionally uninvolved" too far.

You can ask yourself, what might I do to enhance my affect and emotional tone with my patients? If you feel you have to hide from your patients and remain reserved and uninvolved with them, ask yourself why. What might you be protecting? Or what message have you received about being a physician? This potent aspect of the healing relationship may have been missing from your side without your ever realizing it. The emerging new paradigm of health care work is going to be much more equalized between professional helpers and those they help. We are all going to be required to ease up and come more from the heart, rather than falling into those superficial roles of "expert" stereotyped behavior.

A good place to begin practicing being more potent in your own expression is to start coming out more expressively with people you feel very comfortable with. You might even talk this over with a close friend or family member and see what feedback you get about your style of communication.

Often, I hear horror stories about how rude or arrogant a doctor has been with their patients and family members. I'm sure you hear this as well. My son is a long-time juvenile diabetic and more recent kidney transplant patient. So we've had many doctors in our lives for over thirty years—ever since he was two years old. I've had the experience of being completely ignored and "looked through as though I don't exist" by doctors and hospital personnel who know I'm the mother and main caregiver for my son. And we also have doctors, nurses, and other medical helpers, such as EMS technicians, who take the time to really listen and appear vitally interested in my son and respectful of our family members. In today's medical milieu, it's been all over the page. And part of this is the dysfunctional system itself.

Often, a doctor's level of success with his patients is a matter of being high or low in Potency. And sometimes, just making this simple awareness conscious will help remedy it. We all have an inherent ability to be compassionate and personable with one another. So the question becomes, why aren't we willing? Perhaps some big illusion is in the way. Food for thought!

Remember, though, this quality is measuring a *being level* characteristic; it is not a skill that can simply be picked up with practice. If you're low in Potency, you may need to do some personal work on yourself. Something from your childhood or your past may be following you through your life like an unwanted ghost, keeping you from believing in yourself, and causing you to miss out on having a passionate, enlivened response to others and in all areas of your life.

# Chapter Ten

# Self-Actualization

DEFINITION: Enjoying relative independence and self-suffi-
ciency. Being one's authentic self with a broad-minded
attitude toward others. Self-actualization is a result of
advanced personal, emotional, mental, and philosophical or spiritual development. It can be defined as an
individuated personality.

DESCRIPTION: Self-actualization is not merely a trait or characteristic—it is a description of the whole person in the
process of living fully in life as oneself, encompassing
all the other nine personality variables, which correlate
with being an authentic helper.

The word "self-actualization" was coined by Abraham
Maslow, who found there are two kinds of people in the world—
those who are invested in maximizing or actualizing their whole
selfhood, and those who live by society's or the outer world's
standards only. Self-actualization is actually a technical term
whose definition is based on Abraham Maslow's scientific
research. It measures a person's willingness to forget poses, defenses
and shyness and go "whole-hog" into being one's authentic self.

Self-actualizers seek out growth choices rather than becoming enmeshed in society's ways in an unthinking manner.

Self-actualizers learn by looking within, making a strong alignment with their essential Self, their true essence. Non-actualizers learn from looking outside themselves at what they are supposed to be and strive to live up to others' standards, formulas, and ideals. Becoming inner directed will naturally lead to self-actualization, because inner work always leads us to the true Self who lives within each of us as our center, or core identity.

According to Dr. Maslow, self-actualizers live from positive values he called B-values, meaning values of being, rather than from reacting to ego-deficiency needs for safety, emotional highs, or self-acceptance through comparison with others. High-level positive B-values are ultimate values that are intrinsic to our nature. They cannot be reduced to anything more ultimate. They are the qualities we call "soul qualities" in our work, such as goodness, beauty, truth, and acceptance of what *is*.

For example, a self-actualizer would seek out the truth or goodness in a situation per se rather than by gaining validation from society's accepted standards and rules. Their ethics may actually vary according to the particular situation. They have integrated egos, meaning they live beyond the need for much ego gratification due to their high level of emotional health and self-acceptance.

Self-actualized people do not fear living from the heart, being open and receptive to others in ways that encourage equality in relationship. And they have a willingness to always own their own part in any troublesome disagreement or breakdown in communication. We feel very comfortable in relation to self-actualizers because they are open-minded and non-judgmental. They realize everyone has the right to make their own mistakes and to learn from their own experience what life is all about. And they are very clear that everyone makes mistakes!

They experience life fully, vividly, selflessly, with full concentration and total absorption, with little or no self-consciousness. They are wholly and fully human. Or you might say the self-actualization process is an ongoing process of becoming more and more of the whole Self.

Self-actualizers live more in the moment. They have resolved most of their family-of-origin issues and no longer live by others' ideas of right and wrong, but more from their own experienced realizations about what's loving and unloving in life. They think for themselves and are not dependent on others for self-validation. Yet, they rarely feel they need to "lay their philosophies and beliefs" on others. Self-actualizers are basically emotionally healthy. When personal problems are encountered, they will avoid denial and seek solutions, often with the help of others.

When a person begins self-actualizing, values are shifted and sometimes lifestyles become obsolete or a person will go back to school to study for an entirely new profession. Often, this can create a transformational crisis in one's life. We see this constantly in our work. Self-actualizers continually work on themselves when they feel a need for emotional healing or for being with a community of like-minded souls. They attend workshops and undergo various forms of therapy, never feeling like they "have arrived."

Self-actualizing therapists or physicians are not concerned with teaching or lecturing as though they are experts on others. They are much more concerned with helping their patients realize their own wisdom and unique style of being in the world, although this indirect approach takes time that is difficult to find in today's medical model of pharmeucitical and cognitive behavioristic methodologies.

People who are self-actualizers see the extra-ordinary in the ordinary, and have "peak" experiences—often considered mystical or religious subjective experiences. These potent inner experiences are life changing events, sometimes referred to as a conversion or total transformation. This does not apply to everyone who is a self-actualizer, though. There tend to be two types: the mystical and the customary, generally accepted thinker. In other words, you can be a self-actualizer without having a "mystical bent" or a seeker of the extraordinary.

Physicians who are self-actualizers do not function in cold, aloof, distancing ways with their patients. They don't operate out of the fear of being known, or of being sued. They come more from the heart, and from a willingness to just be themselves in relation to their patients. They have no need to be seen as "the expert," or the one who is to maintain the ultimate authority on one's healing process. They are open-minded, willing to listen and respect their patients' own wisdom and needs. They are potent and possessors of great wisdom and knowledge about their practice, but they have no need to behave as though they are superior. They often have quite a bit of humility instead.

Self-actualizing doctors rarely, if ever, get sued! And why? Because their patients feel emotionally close to them, and have no need to find fault with them, even if they make a serious clinical error. This statement is based on the general idea behind the research that's coming out now about the types of doctors who do get sued (5).

Here are some comparisons in how a self-actualizing physician and a non-actualizing physician might sound:

**Self-actualization-in-action:**

Doctor: It's good to see you, Laura. It's been awhile.

Laura: Well, I've come for some advice, I suppose. I'm about to have a nervous breakdown, and I may just need some of your kind words, or perhaps some medication to at least help me sleep.

Doctor: What's going on?

Laura: I've fallen in love with another man. And Robert doesn't know. I'm miserable and feel like a dishonest person. And I don't want to hurt him. He's such a good man. But this is happening to me, and I can't seem to help the feelings that I have. You probably know that Robert's and my marriage has really been dead now for years. We've just never done anything about it.

Doctor: Well, golly, Laura. I can just imagine how split and confused you must feel. To me, this is one of those tragedies that happens in life where we don't intend to harm anyone, but someone does always get hurt. I really feel for you. How can I help with this? And who is this new man in your life?

The doctor is being completely honest, with no superficial responses or any need to guilt her. He's simply being there for her, very real and open, and willing to be of help. He may even have a value system totally opposed to what she is getting herself into. Adultery? Divorce? But he's not laying his trip on her at all, because he knows she has the right to live her own life in her own way.

### Here's another example:

Patient: Hello, Doctor Vasquez. It's so good to finally get here! I've gotten so off-track in my life, I feel like I'm coming apart.

Doctor: What's happening with you, Jimmy? I can see that you're looking awfully pale, and you've lost a lot of weight.

Patient: Well, I've walked out on the church. And my wife is having a holy fit about it. I can't stand our religion anymore and just can't handle being around these people who talk about The Lord all the time and are so d——— judgmental of anyone who doesn't believe exactly as they do. To me, it has just become disgusting. I can't live this kind of lie anymore. And I'm afraid it's going to ruin my marriage. My digestive system is so screwed up, I can't even keep food on my stomach. And besides, I could be wrong. Maybe I'm going to burn in hell. This is truly a God-awful crisis for me, doc.

Doctor: Wow! Jimmy. It sounds like you are beginning to think for yourself, but are having real trouble believing what you think. . . or that it's even okay to think for yourself. Is that right?

Patient: That's it! I'm finding that "my religion" isn't fitting anymore with what I see as reality. It seems to be violating the principles that rule our "oh so very human nature." And. . . if God didn't want us to be human, why would He have made us human? I just can't put it together anymore.

Doctor: Well, I honor you for no longer living in blind faith. I'm not here to tell you how to believe. But I can sure support you while you search for a spiritual life that really feeds you. I do know some very good books on this subject. Would that help? And I certainly know I can help you get your digestive track back in line. So let's talk awhile.

**Toxic Responses:**

In the first example:

Doctor: Fallen in love with another man? My gosh, have you *slept* with him? And you're still married to Robert? How on earth has this happened? Surely you know this isn't right. Some people would even say you're living in sin.

This response is judgmental and guilting. And coming from an authority figure like someone's physician, it carries a lot of weight and could even lead this woman to a deep, deep depression or even suicide. Even if what she is doing violates the doctor's own value system or religious beliefs, as a professional helper, he need not "lay his trip" on his patient. This would be as immoral as he believes she is being by "committing adultery."

In the second example:

Doctor: What do you mean you've left your church? How can you walk out on what the Bible says is true? Remember, the Bible is God's word.

This is a close-minded, guilting statement that doesn't give the patient a chance to talk about what's happened with him. It's as though the doctor has already decided his fate—which is apparently to burn in hellfire and damnation.

Or another toxic response from a non-actualizer would sound like this:

Doctor: So you've lost your spirituality, have you? Well, tell me. What have you been doing that would cause you to get so lost? Sounds to me like you're getting awfully confused.

This statement gives no thought of how this crisis might be leading this patient into a whole new way of knowing God, or of being spiritual. It is a close-minded response based in society's standards of what spirituality is supposed to look like.

A self-actualizing doctor will not behave as though she has all the answers. And she will leave one's ways of being "moral" and "spiritual" to each patient. She will be very willing to listen, to have compassion for what her patients are going through, but she will never be judgmental or "preachy" about how the person ought to live their lives. She may listen for any kind of physical or emotional help she might be able to offer as a physician. Or, she might recommend the patient see a therapist or some other type of health practitioner to help give relief from the stress—body work, acupuncture, personal growth workshops, herbal supplements, things like that.

Non-actualizing physicians won't know how to keep an open mind about such matters as these mentioned above by these two patients. They will either be just followers of the norm with unexamined belief systems thoroughly in place. Or, they might belong to a religious or philosophical school of thought that judges these patients as being immoral or "sinners".

Self-actualizers can have strong belief systems themselves, and can even be part of a certain religion or have a church-going life. But they will never feel like they need to tell others how to live. They will always see the beauty in one's own search for the truth and never behave as though they have all the answers. They know much of life is lived in the gray areas, rather than in extreme black and white. Living life, to them, is living in the mystery. And they are not only comfortable with this very realistic "state of unknowing;" they welcome it.

### Self-reflection:

Becoming self-actualized is a life-long process. It could even be a process that unfolds through many lifetimes! Who knows? Ask yourself: How rigid have you become in how you view philosophical and religious issues concerning life's meaning and our connection to a Higher Power? How open-minded can you realistically be?

And as a physician, how rigid have you become in the existing medical model paradigm? Self-actualizers see that frankly our medical system is currently in a process of a badly needed transformation and expansion into more integrative ways of providing physical health care. You may not have noticed that spirituality and science are merging today to bring us a whole new paradigm of holistic health care. This means you may need to "die" to some of your old ways of thinking and open to new ways that are still unfamiliar to you.

If you feel you have become dogmatic, rigid, or judgmental, ask yourself how come? Are you coming from fear? Are you just following your family chain of how it's always been? Do you think for yourself? Are you able to say "I don't know?" Do you ever question whether or not your beliefs really track with human nature and life as it is? Are you willing to "live the mystery," knowing that we can never know, but we can choose a doctrine of beliefs that contain the qualities of compassion and divine love for all of humanity, regardless of our differences.

With the paradigm shifts occurring all around us today, this is a good chapter to end with: knowing that we may all be called to self-actualize into our next right step on the ladder of human evolution. Human psychology and medicine are changing, because human beings are! Your patients are not the same as they once were. Many are baby-boomers who do think for themselves. And complementary or integrative medicine are no longer on the fringes; they are becoming mainstream very rapidly now (10). So you may be called to seek better and better ways to prevent and treat disease, including any of your own that may be in the way of your own growth and transformation.

I certainly know that if you've read this far, you are indeed a seeker of truth, and a willing participant in learning to marry your mind with your heart. In this regard, may the information in this book help you become more whole.

# EPILOGUE

It is my hope that traveling through these pages has enabled you to see yourself on every page with utter self-honesty. And hopefully, in all the positive ways you are already there for your patients, regardless of how similar or different they may be from you and how you live your life.

Improving your bedside manner, though, will always be a relevant issue for those of you in the medical world. It will always lead you to more and more good self-feeling and love for your chosen profession. You will remember that you came into the medical profession because you want to save lives and help people who are suffering. You will remember that this is your chosen life's work that truly gives your life meaning and a strong sense of purpose.

Now that you've studied all 10 of these personality variables that correlate with effective helping, you are no doubt seeing that they don't operate in isolation; they all fit together as one way of being with your clients, as one attitude about life and helping others.

There is a story about the centipede that was crossing the street, her hundred legs flowing gracefully in perfect symmetry, moving her along with perfect ease.

A little girl noticed this amazing creature with all these legs. And, in awe, she asked, "How are you doing this? How are you keeping all those legs working together like that?"

The centipede stopped, looked down at her legs, tried to analyze how she was doing this, walked some more, and fell all over herself, her legs all tangled up in a knot.

———

We don't want to analyze ourselves too much, or try to work too hard at becoming *naturally* therapeutic. It's better to just go about your business, willing to note the traits you are strong in and the ones where you might need a little work. Then, anytime you start to feel your conversations with a patient running amok, you can reflect on what you've read here, and discover which trait you are void in. Every difficulty in communicating will be an absence of one of these traits!

And learn to trust your natural style of listening and "being there" for your patients. If you are the soft, easy-going type of helper, you'll probably be best at establishing rapport with your patients. If you are more reserved and structured in your way of being, you may be better at the more disciplined, challenging ways of relating to your patients. Either way can be therapeutic, and your natural style can also be balanced by practicing the traits that don't come as naturally for you.

Just remember that recognizing and honoring the good in yourself, as well as the good in all you serve, is love made visible! And hopefully, we're all entering into a whole new paradigm of medical and mental health care that can more easily "come from the heart."

# References

(1) See Truax, C.B. and Carkhuff, R.R., *Toward Effective Counseling and Psychotherapy: Training and Practice.* Chicago: Aldine Publishing Company, 1967. See also the work of Sidney Wolf, *An Investigation of Counselor Type, Client Type, Level of Facilitative Conditions and Client Outcome,* Catholic University of America, Dissertation Abstracts International, 1970, 31, Order No. 70-22,093. And his ADPA Paper entitled *"Counseling for Better or for Worse,"* 23rd Annual Meeting, September 10-15, 1972, Atlanta, Georgia.

(2) See Starfield, Barbara. "Is the U.S. Health Really Best in the World?" *Journal of American Medical Association*, Vol. 284, No. 4, July 26,2000, pp. 483-485. See also, Hoffman, Ronald F., M.D. with Stevens, Sidney. *How to Talk to Your Doctor,* Basic Health Publications, Inc., Laguna Beach, CA, 2006.

(3) *The New York Times*, "Health Fitness,"Tuesday, June 1, 2004.

(4) Gladwell, Malcolm, *Blink, The Power of Thinking Without Thinking,* Little, Brown and Company, NY, 2005, pp. 41-43.

(5) *American-Statesman, Austin*, November 30, 2005, pp. A-1 and A-9, entitled "In patient care, empathy is the RX for ill manners, doctors learn," by Gina Kolata, *New York Times*.

(6) Pert, Candace B., *Molecules of Emotion,* NY, Scribner, 1997

(7) See *Newsweek Magazine*, September 27, 2004, and *Time Magazine*, January 17, 2005, for full reports on this subject.

(8) Adapted from The Harvard Medical School Mental Health Letter. For more information, go to health.Harvard.edu/newsweek.

(9) "We All Need a Dose of the Doctor," *Newsweek Magazine*, Sepbember 27, 2004, page 64.

(10) Hoffman, Ronald L. and Stevens, Sidney, *How to Talk to Your Doctor*, Basic Health Publications, Inc., Laguna Beach, CA, 2006.

# About the Authors

Jacquelyn Small, LMSW, is a Phi Beta Kappa graduate of the University of Texas at Austin with degrees in Psychology and Clinical Social Work. She is widely recognized in the field of psychotherapy training and the author of the classic *Becoming Naturally Therapeutic*, widely used in many university and agency settings for training in psychotherapy. She has served on the adjunct faculty of the Institute of Transpersonal Psychology and as the Clinical Director for the Texas Commission on Alcoholism and Drug Abuse, and teaches in many health care and continuing education settings nationally. Jacquelyn is the Founder of the Eupsychia Institute, a non-profit service provider in counselor healing and training. Jacquelyn is the author of nine books on personal growth.

Jim Mulry, MD has practiced family medicine for 30 years. He taught family practice at a midwest medical school and is certified in addictionology, medical acupuncture, and The Eupsychia Process of Psychospiritual Integration and Integrative Breathwork.

OTHER BOOKS BY JACQUELYN SMALL,
AVAILABLE THROUGH EUPSYCHIA INSTITUTE:

*Becoming Naturally Therapeutic*
Bantam, 1992

*Transformers, the Therapists of the Future*
DeVorss & Co., 1982; Bantam, 1992

*Awakening in Time:*
*The Journey from Co-dependence to Co-creation*
Bantam, 1993

*Embodying Spirit: Coming Alive with Meaning and Purpose*
HarperSanFrancisco, 1994

*Living Your Bigger Story: The Practice of Self-Remembrance*
Hazelden, 1995

*Rising to the Call: A Handbook for Evolving Souls*
(with Mary Yovino)
DeVorss & Co., 1997

*Becoming A Practical Mystic*
Quest Books, 1998

*Psyche's Seeds: The 12 Principles of Soul-based Psychology*
Tarcher/Putnam, 2001

*The Sacred Purpose of Being Human*
Health Communications, 2005

Jacquelyn Small is available to conduct trainings
for a variety of medical providers, educators
and organizations interested in
*Improving Your Bedside Manner.*

Contact Brenda Shea at Eupsychia
for more information:

Brenda Shea
Eupsychia Institute
PO Box 151960
Austin, TX 78715-1960
800-546-2795
eupsychia@austin.rr.com
www.ImprovingYourBedsideManner.com